Introduction

Our immune system is dependent upon minerals and vitamins that are absorbed into your body naturally and these nutrients have been produced over time starting at the bottom of the sea after at the moment of the big bang evolved in our planet and within us at the moment of conception. We are created and nature is created for us and into the garden of Eden we can return for the natural health as our creator has given.

This is energy that is the universal connection from the micro-world to macro-world of an ever expanding universe that spans billions of miles and billions of years in a perfect balance of energy in a time and space continuum. Variance in this nature will adjust to reestablish balance with trillions of bacteria and cellular activity for the survival of the fittest. This is a metamorphosis of constant evolution from the oceans where we came.

From the depths of the ocean floor where volcanic towers that form the earth's crust aquatic creatures exist in multitudes. Deep at the molten center core of our planet nutrition began. Here the heavy metals are formed in towers of volcanic metals are fed upon by six foot aquatic worms that use bacteria to chemically synthesize nutrition for life. Here the nutrition is created from heavy metals into soft metals for consumption of plants by organisms that rose from the sea and salt to house in their body a chemical electrical system of mineral and vitamin based metabolic functioning for energy that is the constant metamorphosis of the entire universe. The fish have central nervous system and eye vision just like us from mineral nutrition and nature has stem cells for creating the body. Some of the metamorphic functions are called stem cells and at the surface of our body are Astrocytes or Star Cells that regenerate skin. It mirrors the galaxy on a micro scale what is in the stars that are above and are connected through a stem cell universe within the trillion connections of our Central Nervous System in a chemical electrical saltwater solution. This stem cell system was started at the moment of our conception that is natural and it stems out words from what they call the Super Cell and like a conductor, direct a symphony of our body and mind constructing our body and mind.

Here in the essence of ourselves we are united by nourishment and growth and in life our union of the body and mind with nourishment is the most important choice we make for our health and wellbeing. This nutritive connection that was formed so we could consume to produce our body is the key to mental and physical wellness. Disease of all sorts are dependent upon our nutrition to heal.

It is the mission of this book to show that nutrition, solar radiation, oxygen and aerobic respiration is the power of nature and that we possess the power through minerals and vitamins within the plant system that has evolved over time to create a body and mind from the moment of conception they call a Zygote and I call the energy of your first breath.

As our first growth established gastro intestinal feeding to eat so our stem cells formed with a blueprint of DNA the primal force of feeding for survival was passed from our ancestors. Here in a small bang of energy the chemical synthesis from your parents aided with reproductive stem cells of your mother started a sprouting forming all of your body. As we travel through time and space we are aided by the energy of the radiant Sun and the Oxygen to breathe and the nutrition that are the three pillars of healthy life that is disease free and the healing power of creation which is metamorphosis, the power of natural healing. Aerobic exercise from work or regimen motivate the pillars for integrity of structure.

The entire universe is a constant state of metamorphosis into energy from the consumption and production of nutrients powered by the radiation of the sun and billions of years of mother nature have created a perfect balance of plants and animals that produce, consume and energize. This system or process is the most powerful and is the subject of research to leash this power. To upset this with scientific modeling will force mother nature to mutate to counteract the chemical attack on the natural process. Science is the study of nature by definition and mother nature took billions of years to evolve in a perfect balance of life and nutrition to maintain and sustain life.

The only way to fight the chemical attack is to eat as close as possible organic foods for nutrition, use breath control to maximize oxygen and exercise so the radiated nutrients heat up for chemical transfer which is metamorphosis into energy and

purity for health and wellbeing. There is no man made pill or invention that is superior to this.

We were born with this process and our spiritual power rises as we energize from enlightenment into Christ Consciousness where we are one with universe that is energy. This is the miracle of life given to us by creation.

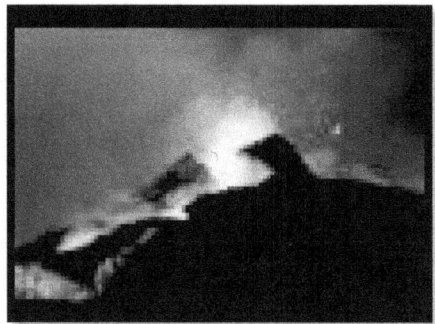

Here in the ocean nutrition began from the pure molten rock and the aquatic life used bacteria to convert the heavy metals into nutrition that is biological degradable in our body.

.

Many things have been said about mineral salt baths and the healing power of this. People flock to these because the water is filled with minerals that have been purified in the earth's core, chemically synthesized into nutritional fuel for our metabolic function.

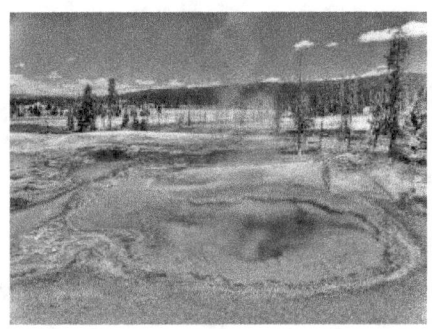

The earth's core distributes minerals for planet energy and healing power in a survival for the fittest. From the depths of the ocean to our table for eating, the mineral food chain is the most powerful energy producing light that is Einstein formula, Energy = Mass x The Speed of Light Squared. Within and without us this light travels and this power is second to none when it comes to healing. This light travels through our body and binds to matter that is the mineral compound of health and wellbeing.

Chapter 1 Nutrition of the Sea and Sun

Within our body there is a universe of trillions of transmissions energized by metabolism that regenerates our cells from conception and our entire life. Nourished, the stem cell structure built our body and continues to protect and aid in health and wellbeing. From the early fertilization the animal cells are nourished by the vegetal cells that create the energy of metamorphosis and the harmony of nutrition and energy that builds a human being. This phenomenal creative power will never be replicated and it took millions of years to form who we are and all of nature was involved. In the depths of the sea bacteria aids aquatic life upon towering volcanic formations that are 600 degrees hot to chemically transfer heavy metals into nutrition of iron, manganese and calcium into soft palatable food filled with nutritive benefits that fuel the regeneration enduring our lives **"Hilário, of Portugal's University of Aveiro, and colleagues recently found 20 species of the tiny worms, called frenulates, in mud volcanoes in the Gulf of Cádiz, an arm of the Atlantic Ocean southwest of Spain.**

Mud volcanoes are places where methane-filled fluids seep from the seafloor, providing energy for "exceptionally rich ecosystems," Hilário said in an email.

But scientists know little about the elusive frenulates, tube-dwelling worms that survive thanks to bacteria that live inside a special organ in their bodies.

The worms absorb chemicals such as methane from sediment and deliver the substances, via their blood, to the bacteria, which in turn produce organic carbon. The carbon nourishes both creatures."

Hilario has already named another genus from the expedition Bobmarleya—the worm's "dreadlocked" appearance reminded her of the Jamaican singer, she said.

—Christine Dell'Amore

Photograph courtesy Ana Hilário

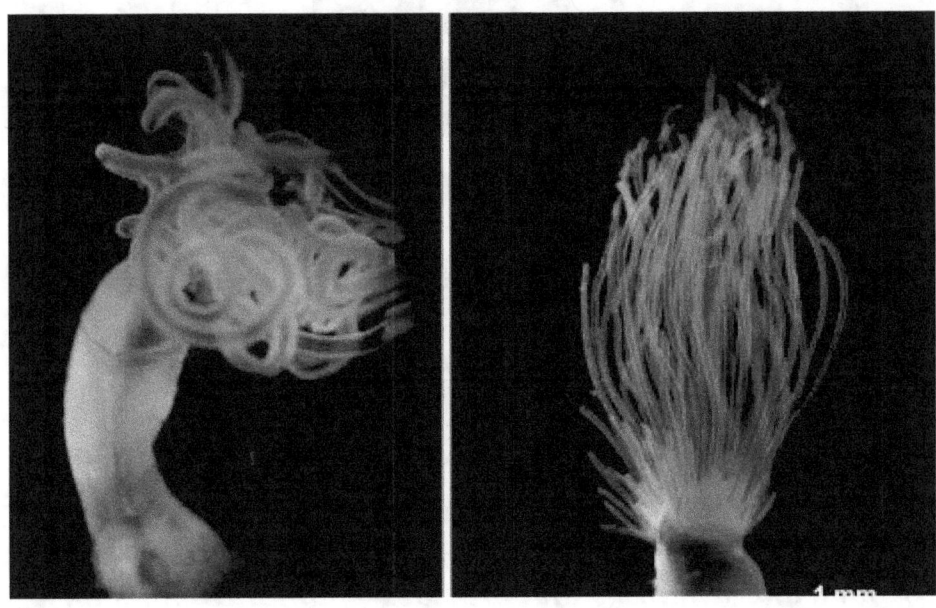

1 mm

In the depths of the ocean where the plates of continents separate the earth's core begins the nutritional food chain of the crust to the earth's garden. This mineral rich offering sits still while we are mobile to pick the fruits of the paradise and greens of the forest that breathes with radiation of the sun as we do. There are three important natural healing aids that maintain health. They are the radiation of the sun, the oxygen that breaks down matter for energy and the nutritive minerals and vitamins that is the fuel of the universe to generate energy.

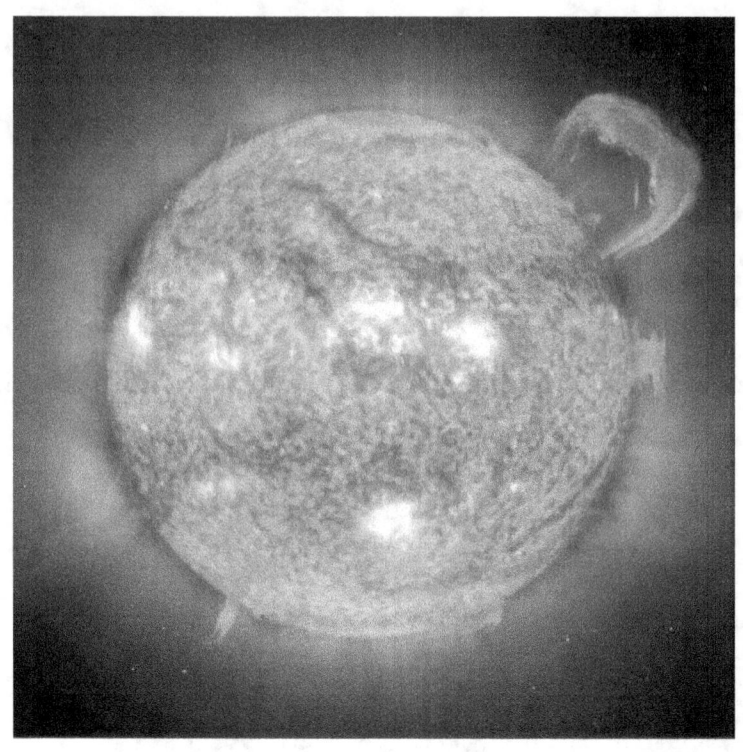

Radiation is the emission of energy through waves of light through space in all direction as the Sun does. From this we and the plants soak in this for energy to grow.

*The Sun helps the creation of food and within us that provides Vitamin D that binds to intestinal absorption of calcium, iron, magnesium, manganese, phosphate and zinc that are proteins or molecular sugars. These minerals create in a chemical synthesis a metamorphosis of immune fighting power of enzymes **that** protect you from disease. This is a product of lymphocytes that are produced by the Lymph Glands that fight infection. Here they create, in your bloodstream, immune strength.*

The heat of the sun causes chemical reactions throughout our planet that give rise to life. The study of physics is the study of nature and we are part of nature the mobile part that depend on this link for immune strength. The chemical synthesis that is a metamorphosis of life and tissue needs heat or aerobic respiration to allow oxygen to break down and through consumption on nutrients to the production of polymers and steroids plus much more. Comparatively, when we cook and put spices for taste the heat warms the sauce and the chemical transfer occurs making the sauce spicy. This is what your body goes through to spice up your blood. So it is necessary to use the sun radiation and additional activity to chemical transfer the minerals for health.

Vitamin D binds with Amino acids that are proteins. The proteins are production from the consumption of minerals and are synthesized into sugars of molecular value that uses the radiated vitamins to fight disease. When plants bear fruit they use the radiation of the sun in photosynthesis and when ripened have natural sugars that are ready as nutrition. We ripen internally for the natural sugars to be joined with Sun radiation to create immune defenses that neutralize disease and bodily malfunctions.

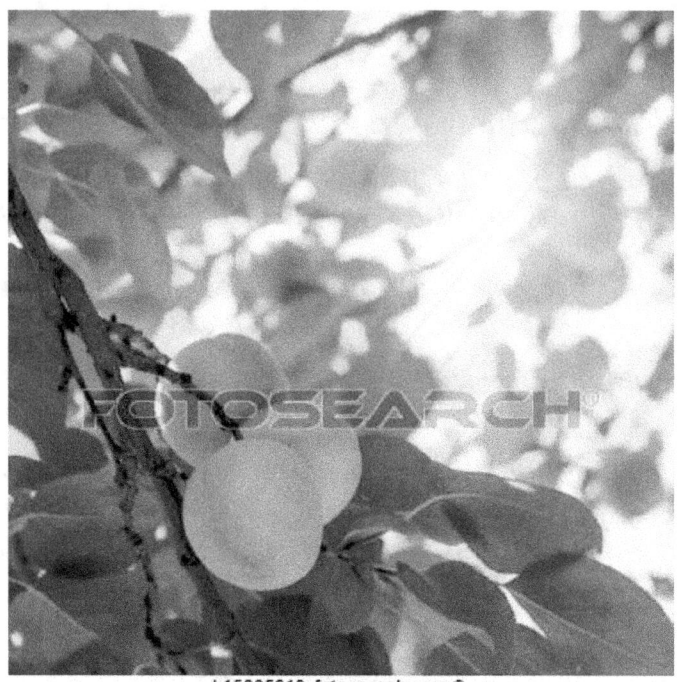

"Vitamin D is carried in the bloodstream to the liver, where it is converted into the prohormone calcidiol (The first step in the oxidative degradation of organic compounds). Circulating calcidiol may then be converted into calcitriol, the biologically active form of vitamin D, in the kidneys. Following the final converting step in the kidney, calcitriol is released into the circulation. By binding to vitamin D-binding protein, a carrier protein in the plasma, calcitriol is transported to various target organs. About Vitamin D". University of California, Riverside. November 2011. Retrieved January 24, 2015. *In addition to the kidneys, calcitriol is also synthesized by monocyte-macrophages (single cell-big eaters) in the immune system. When synthesized by monocyte-macrophages, calcitriol acts locally as a cytokine (cell signaling), defending the body against microbial invaders by stimulating the innate immune system."* Adams

JS, Hewison M; Hewison (2010). "Update in Vitamin D". Journal of Clinical Endocrinology & Metabolism 95 (2): 471–8. doi:10.1210/jc.2009-1773. PMC 2840860. PMID 20133466

The full process of solar radiation for the oxygen breakdown of organic compounds lasts 7 days and the need to have 20 minutes of unfiltered sunlight will supply the body with immune power and without it deficiency levels will suppress immune building functions. The circulation of the vitamins that are degraded into organic compounds reach the gut through the filtering of the liver and kidneys to place needed compounds for your health and wellbeing. The entire universe is the constant creation of energy through breakdown of oxygen that is from fresh nutrients that ripen and synthesize into energy.

"A systematic clinical studies shows an association between low vitamin D levels, cognitive impairment, and a higher risk of developing Alzheimer's disease. However, lower vitamin D concentrations is also associated with poor nutrition and spending less time outdoors. Therefore, alternative explanations for the increase in cognitive impairment exist and hence a direct causal relationship between vitamin D levels and cognition could not be established review of." Balion C, Griffith LE, Strifler L, Henderson M, Patterson C, Heckman G, Llewellyn DJ, Raina P (2012). "Vitamin D, cognition, and dementia: a systematic review and meta-analysis". Neurology 79 (13): 1397–405. doi:10.1212/WNL.0b013e31826c197f. PMC 3448747. PMID 23008220. I dki

The vital role of radiation as the synthesized sunlight defends us in a biochemical process with hydration and oxygen to defend and eliminate toxins and fight cancer, flu, asthma and many more attacks upon our immune system to suppress our immunity. This is how our immune system is activated and arms our lymph gland. This arming is the distribution of Macro phage or big eaters into the bloodstream from lymph glands that are the neutralizing disease that are cell killing of diseases that are cells sending disease through our bloodstream. The diseases send out Nagalese that will neutralize the Macro Phages. Mineral strength will win the battle but mineral weakness will allow disease to establish and grow. Mineral deficiency is a major problem with our food and water and is the cause of many ailments.

"Vitamin D supplements have been widely marketed for their claimed anticancer properties. Associations have been shown in observational studies between low vitamin D levels and the risk of development of certain cancers including colon cancer." Ma, Y; Zhang, P; Wang, F; Yang, J; Liu, Z; Qin, H (1 October 2011). "Association between vitamin D and risk of colorectal cancer: a systematic review of prospective studies.". Journal of clinical oncology : official journal of the American Society of Clinical Oncology 29 (28): 3775–82. PMID 21876081

"The universe is swamped in neutrinos that are left over from the Big Bang, and many more are created in nuclear reactions on earth and in the thermonuclear reactions that power the sun."

Once thought to be massless and to travel at the speed of light, they drift through the earth and our own bodies like moonlight through a window. Knowing that they can change identities means that they have mass, and that has helped cosmologists understand how the universe has evolved and how the sun works and perhaps will help them improve their attempts to create fusion reactors on earth."

http://www.nytimes.com/2015/10/07/science/nobel-prize-physics

"Neutrinos do not carry any electric charge, which means that they are not affected by the electromagnetic force that acts on charged particles, and are leptons, so they are not affected by the strong force that acts on particles inside atomic nuclei. Neutrinos are therefore affected only by the weak subatomic force and by gravity. The weak force is a very short-range interaction, and gravity is extremely weak on the subatomic scale. Thus, neutrinos typically pass through normal matter unimpeded and undetected." https://en.wikipedia.org/wiki/Neutrino

Like moonlight through glass it carries the space into us and has matter. What an incredible magic in our body and this it tied into the radiant energy of the sun. This is the path of healing that is interconnected within and without us. The sun and its radiant power help construct energy for immunity. This will help us understand the not only how to leash the power of thermonuclear power of the sun but that this is the power of nature that combines with the planet and all who inhabit it as a nuclear reaction for immune defenses and the energy it produces is the energy of one world connection. In my first book Yoga Light I talk about Kundalini Chakras or energy centers and the neutrinos information can help understand the power of meditation. From this phenomenon we are connected physically on the molecular level to the sun and we are part of nature that is the power of healing. Within and without us is this floating energy that is not charged and radiate throughout the universe. The radiation of this power enters our body as non-electric and metamorphose into mass and binds to the minerals that it energized to grow coming in a circle of balance. The efficiency of this movement is the immune system in tune and perfect tuning is a healing power that is a chemical electrical phenomenon. Here is the scientific research about how this phenomenon is tangible and arms our immunity. The molecular compounds from nutrition and solar energy are released in the bloodstream and are big eaters with protein sugars or Gc-maf that devour disease and neutralize the enemy and this is health. The minerals change into amino acids that are natural sugars ripening bind in a compound with the suns radiated energy and like a plant produce immune zapping energy of rotting cells that are trying to grow with an adverse protein that is started from toxins in the body that are numerous including preservatives (heavy metals) and high fructose corn syrup (manipulated sugars). These proteins fight for turf in the blood stream and the fittest one wins the battle that can be defeat or to succumb to the disease. With the immune strength of minerals and sunlight we can defeat disease but if the rotting cells are fed with toxins we will lose the survival of the fittest. This is explained in science for your reference.

"Biochemically, Gc-MAF results from sequential deglycosylation of the vitamin D-binding protein (the Gc protein), which is naturally promoted by lymphocytes (B and

T cells). The resulting protein may be a macrophage activating factor (MAF).[1] *MAFs are lymphokines that control the expression of antigens on the surface of macrophages, and one of their functions is to make macrophages become cytotoxic (cell killing) to tumors. Gc-MAF may play a role in various diseases"* Malik, Suneil; Fu, Lei; Juras, David James; Karmali, Mohamed; Wong, Betty Y. L.; Gozdzik, Agnes; Cole, David E. C. (January–February 2013). "Common variants of the vitamin D binding protein gene and adverse health outcomes". *Critical Reviews in Clinical Laboratory Sciences 50 (1): 1–22.doi:10.3109/10408363.2012.750262. PMC 3613945.PMID 23427793.*

The cell killing is what Chemo Therapy does and the radiation of the sun produces cell killing from nuclear reaction that does not have collateral damage kills other cells and is specific to the cancer with sugars of chemical synthesis that is deployed in the body for a direct attack on disease. "Glucose is made during photosynthesis from water and carbon dioxide, using energy from sunlight. The reverse of the photosynthesis reaction(deglycosylation), which releases this energy, is a very important source of power for cellular respiration. Glucose is stored as a polymer, in plants as starch and in animals as glycogen. Use of glucose as an energy source in cells is by either aerobic respiration, anaerobic respiration, or fermentation. All of these processes follow from an earlier metabolic pathway known as glycolysis" http://neuroscience.uth.tmc.edu/s4/chapter11.htm

"Through glycolysis and later in the reactions of the citric acid cycle and oxidative phosphorylation, glucose is oxidized to eventually form CO_2 and water, yielding energy mostly in the form of ATP. The insulin reaction, and other mechanisms,

regulate the concentration of glucose in the blood. Glucose supplies almost all the energy for the brain, so its availability influences psychological processes. When glucose is low, psychological processes requiring mental effort (e.g., self-control, effortful decision-making) are impaired." Fairclough, Stephen H.; Houston, Kim (2004), "A metabolic measure of mental effort" Biol. Psychol. 66 (2): 177–90, doi:10.1016/j.biopsycho.2003.10.001, PMID 15041139.

So we sweeten inside from minerals and vitamins from the sun and plants and produce energy when its breaks down with oxygen. It is a path of health that are the three pillars of immunity that are put into action exercising or working. The plants use the system to produce food loaded with minerals of high nutritional value when they ripen and this process is the same in us. With this energy we rid physical diseases of the body and mind.

The energy that minerals and sunlight gives you is where your brain power is derived. When people constantly eat modified sugars in their food the result is modifies brain activity. Children then in school do not achieve as the parents want and that they could achieve higher planes of understanding and thus making a better world. However, greed places these people in a toxic environment that exploits not the spiritual enlightenment but a retarded and muted energy promoting obesity and mineral deficiency leading to mental and physical diseases.

The three pillars of immunity that form the base of mental and physical health are:

Solar Radiation   *Nutrition*   *Oxygen*

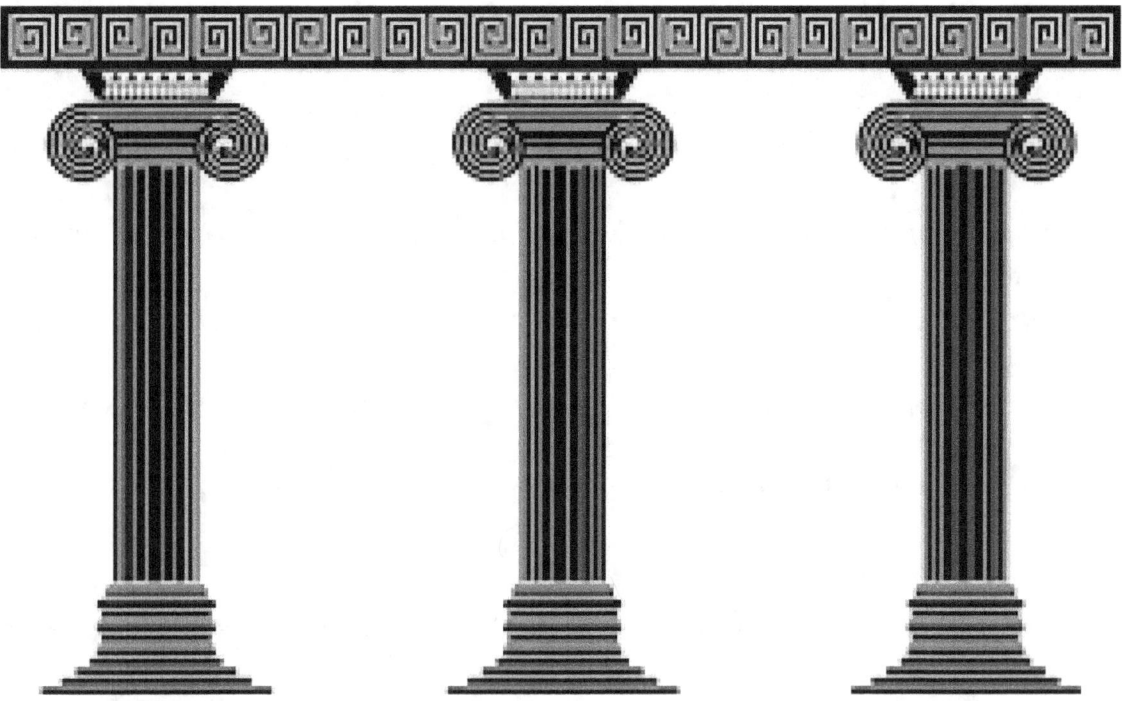

In order to get this energy flowing the movement of oxygen via aerobic exercise and not sedentary behavior that cause the pillars to weaken.

Chapter 2.   Survival of the Fittest

When we are processing with these natural elements we produce cell killing immunity in our bloodstream that removes dead cells that are disease starters. Dead cells produce a rotten protein in our body that tries to overtake our body. This is called Nagalase and the three pillars produce a defender that neutralizes Nagalase called GcMaf. Within your body there is life battle going on that is a protein based offense of diseases and immunity. These sugar based proteins become a survival of the fittest and immunity is produced by the consumption of nutrients and disease is fueled by toxins that both chemically synthesize sugar to energize pathways of healing or dying.

Our body with its immune system uses minerals to metamorphose into disease fighting cells that are cytotoxic or cell killing of cancer cells naturally in a specific attack without damaging a host of healthy cells and the Gc-maf is the cutting edge of healing. Maf is macrophage(Big eaters) and it is a "Gc protein-derived macrophage activating factor is an immunomodulatory protein that, by affecting the immune system, may play a role in various diseases." Malik, Suneil; Fu, Lei; Juras, David James; Karmali, Mohamed; Wong, Betty Y. L.; Gozdzik, Agnes; Cole, David E. C. (January–February 2013) *Macrophages are highly specialized in removal of dying or dead cells and cellular debris. The lack of detoxing allows dead cells to turn into disease and produce Nagalase.*

"What is Nagalase? Nagalase is a protein made by all cancer cells and viruses (HIV, hepatitis B, hepatitis C, influenza, herpes, Epstein-Barr virus, and others). Its formal, official chemical name is alpha-N-acetylgalactosaminidase, but this is such a tongue-twisting mouthful of a moniker that we usually just call it "Nagalase." (Sometimes, when I want to impress friends with my brilliance, I'll say the entire word real fast: "alpha-N-acetylgalactosaminidase." I have found that it's important to practice beforehand if one doesn't want to embarrass oneself.)

Why is Nagalase important?

Nagalase causes immunodeficiency. Nagalase blocks production of GcMAF, thus preventing the immune system from doing its job. Without an active immune system, cancer and viral infections can grow unchecked.

As an extremely sensitive marker for all cancers, Nagalase provides a powerful system for early detection.

Serial Nagalase testing provides a reliable and accurate method for tracking the results of any therapeutic regimen for cancer, AIDS, or other chronic viral infection.

Nagalase proves that cancer cells break all the rules

Normal healthy cells cooperate with one another in a concerted effort to further the good of all. Cancer cells refuse to play ball. Their disdainful attitude toward the rest of our cellular community is appalling. For example, these cellular scofflaws ignore clear messages to stop growing and spreading and encroaching on their neighbor's space. How would you like it if your neighbor moved his fence over into your backyard?

Of all the rules cancer cells break, none is more alarming than the production of Nagalase, the evil enzyme that completely hog-ties the immune system army's ability to stop cancer cells.

Virus particles also make Nagalase. Their goal is the same as that of the cancer cells: survival by incapacitating their number one enemy: the immune system.

Nagalase precision

Like a stealth bomber, the Nagalase enzyme synthesized in and released from a cancer cell or a virus particle pinpoints the GcMAF production facilities on the surface of your T and B lymphocytes and then wipes them out with an incredibly precise bomb. How precise? Let me put it this way: Nagalase locates and attacks one specific two-electron bond located at, and only at, the 420th amino acid position on a huge protein molecule (DBP), one of tens of thousands of proteins, each containing millions of electrons. This is like selectively taking out a park bench in a major city from six thousand miles away. More astonishing, if that is possible, Nagalase never misses its target. There is no collateral damage.

As you already know, GcMAF is a cell-signaling glycoprotein that talks to macrophages, enabling them to rapidly find, attack, and kill viruses and cancer cells. By activating macrophages, GcMAF triggers a cascade that activates the entire immune system. Blockage of GcMAF production by Nagalase brings all this wonderful anti-cancer and anti-viral immune activity to a screeching halt, allowing cancer and infections to spread.

What does Nagalase actually do? How does it destroy immune functioning and deactivate macrophages?

Once synthesized and released into nearby tissue or into the bloodstream, Nagalase, like that drill sergeant at boot camp, shouts harsh commands at the vitamin D binding protein (DBP) that is about to be turned into GcMAF. Nagalase demands that DBP not, under any circumstances, attach itself to a specific sugar molecule (galactosamine). If DBP has already grabbed (i.e., connected to, using a two-electron, "covalent" bond) a galactosamine sugar molecule, it is commanded to immediately let go. "Leave galactosamine alone, or you'll be in big trouble!!!" is the Nagalase sergeant's command. We'll probably never know whether or not, on some deeper level, DBP knows that Nagalase's motives are dastardly—but it doesn't really matter:

DBP will definitely always obey. Like the army private, the DBP literally has no choice. Because of the way hierarchies work in cellular biology, proteins must do the bidding of their enzymes. The enzymes, like Nagalase, are the drill sergeant and the proteins, like DBP, are the privates. That's just the way it is. Obeying the drill sergeant's command means DBP can't do its assigned task, that of becoming GcMAF. It is rendered useless. For DBP, on a molecular level, life no longer has meaning.

Unfortunately for cancer and viral patients, DBP had been on its way to becoming GcMAF until the Nagalase drill sergeant so rudely interrupted. Now GcMAF—the one protein our bodies need in order to activate our immune systems—can't be made. Immune activity screeches to a halt. The defense system protecting us from cancers and viruses has been snuffed out.

Nagalase, using this astonishingly simple yet cunningly subversive technique, emasculates the GcMAF precursor protein (DBP) by knocking off its three sugar molecules. One quick whack by Nagalase and the DBP protein that would have become a GcMAF molecule now limps off into the sunset, permanently disfigured and disabled. With one simple, swift maneuver, Nagalase has brought the entire immune system to its knees.

Here's how Dr. Yamamoto put it (for clarity, I've replaced some of the technical words):

"Serum vitamin D3-binding protein (DBP) is the precursor for the principal macrophage activating factor (GcMAF). The precursor activity of serum DBP was reduced... These patient sera contained alpha-N-acetylgalactosaminidase (Nagalase) that deglycosylates (removes the sugars) DBP. Deglycosylated DBP cannot be converted to GcMAF, thus it loses the GcMAF precursor activity, leading to immunosuppression." (Microbes Infect. 2005 Apr;7(4):674-81. Epub 2005 Mar 22. Pathogenic significance of alpha-N-acetylgalactosaminidase activity found in the hemagglutinin of influenza virus. Yamamoto N, Urade M.)

Nagalase testing: former mass murderer now works for the good guys

It's easy to be a little schizy about Nagalase. On the one hand, this nasty protein's behavior toward us has been reprehensible and disastrous. Working in cahoots with cancer and HIV—not shy about getting into bed with our mortal enemies—Nagalase can rightfully claim direct responsibility for billions of human deaths. And it would just as soon add you to the list, so we don't have to be shy about placing Nagalase in the "genocidal murderer" column.

With the advent of Nagalase testing, however, this bad actor now will be harnessed to a useful purpose. By providing us with precise and reliable advance information about enemy operations, Nagalase blood level testing becomes a "Deep Throat" double agent for cancer. He helps us by giving us an early warning sign.

Early detection (using AMAS or Nagalase) saves lives

You don't want a cancer to have gotten out of control by the time you find and start treating it. When cancers are still young and small, gentle natural therapies are the most effective. Alternative treatments work best on early small cancers by enhancing immune functioning and removing the source of the inflammation that is causing the cancer in the first place. Cancers that have become large enough to see on imaging pose a much more significant threat, and the big guns now become necessary.

*The current method for diagnosing most cancers requires us to wait until a mass shows up on imaging (e.g., a mammogram, chest X-ray, or colonoscopy). This approach wastes valuable time and causes needless deaths. But long before imaging can find it, a positive Nagalase (or **AMAS test**) can tell us that early stage cancer exists somewhere in the body. By enabling earlier and therefore less invasive treatment options, this information provides a huge head-start.*

Normally present at only trace levels, Nagalase shows up in the blood when a cancer or virus appears

The malignant and viral entities that make Nagalase are not normally present, so its appearance is a big deal from a diagnostic perspective. When Nagalase shows up, even in very small amounts, we have the earliest glimpse of a new cancer or viral infection. The old adage, "Where there's smoke, there's fire" applies here. A positive Nagalase test notifies us that a cancer (or a nasty virus) lurks within.

Nagalase appears in the blood stream when a nascent cancer is just a minute cluster of abnormal cells, long before conventional diagnostic methods can detect it. Through blood testing, we can find this red flag, even when present at exceedingly low levels. Providing us with this early warning sign might not quite qualify Nagalase for the "Good Samaritan" award, but I could go with "extremely useful." Like a rehabilitated criminal on parole, the potential for harm is still there. For now, however, he's staying out of trouble and doing community service. Turn your back and he's a mass murderer again.

Using Nagalase testing to track cancer treatment

Rising Nagalase levels indicate a cancer or virus is growing and spreading. Conversely, Nagalase levels will decrease if the cancer or infection is being effectively destroyed.

Any treatment that lowers cancer cell (or viral numbers) will lower Nagalase levels. Nagalase will, for example, always drop after surgery (whether or not the entire tumor was removed). Chemotherapy and radiation also reduce Nagalase levels. So does

GcMAF. If, after these treatments, the depressed level begins to rise again, this is the warning sign that the cancer was not completely removed, and/or that metastatic disease is hiding out somewhere. With viral infections, increasing Nagalase levels indicate return of the infection.

Consecutive rising Nagalase levels are therefore a red flag, warning us it may be time to entertain new treatment options. Conversely, if levels are going down, stay the course: the cancer or virus is going away.

Flat-earth medicine

Many medical professionals don't feel comfortable with "nonspecific" tests like Nagalase. It drives them nuts to discover that a cancer is lurking somewhere inside without knowing exactly where it is located. "How," they ask, "do you expect me to treat a cancer I can't see? Why, I'm not going to tilt at windmills!" This may be a signal that you need to find a different doctor, perhaps one who works in an alternative cancer clinic. Here you will find highly-trained professionals who understand the concept that cancer is a molecular biological change long before it presents visually (by this I mean becomes viewable on imaging).

When GcMAF becomes available, the answer will be easier: a six month course of weekly 100 ng GcMAF intramuscular injections with monthly Nagalase level tests to follow the Nagalase level as it goes back down to baseline. The cancer can be declared cured, even though it never reached life-threatening proportions. (We have a long way to go before this kind of medical behavior will be commonplace and acceptable. The sooner the better, however.)

Nagalase role "under-appreciated"

Nagalase, arguably our most immunosuppressive protein molecule, poses an enormous threat in terms of cancer perpetuation and viruses' ability to continually defeat us. Yet cancer researchers have not shown any interest in it. (Maybe I'm being a little too generous here; perhaps "clueless" would be more a more accurate depiction.) Why don't they get it that blasting cancer cells into oblivion with chemo and radiation is usually not sufficient to stop advanced disease and does nothing to address the cause: immunosuppression. Even if we ignore for the moment the excessive collateral damage caused by chemo drugs and radiation, the patient also needs—requires—a healthy immune system to finish the job. If we don't revive immune function by disabling Nagalase, the cancers and viruses will just keep roaring back. Restoring immujectsunocompetence by negating the stultifying effect of Nagalase should therefore become a primary research goal." Copyright Timothy J Smith 2010

Macrophage means big eaters that reach out to rid us of disease. In order to survive the body evolved from the radiant sun and oxygen a cleaning process in a chemical electrical system of mineral synthesis that supports immunity. This illustration shows the action that consumes, neutralizes and ejects as waste in a curing process that is the power of natural healing through metamorphosis of disease to health and the energy that we possess.

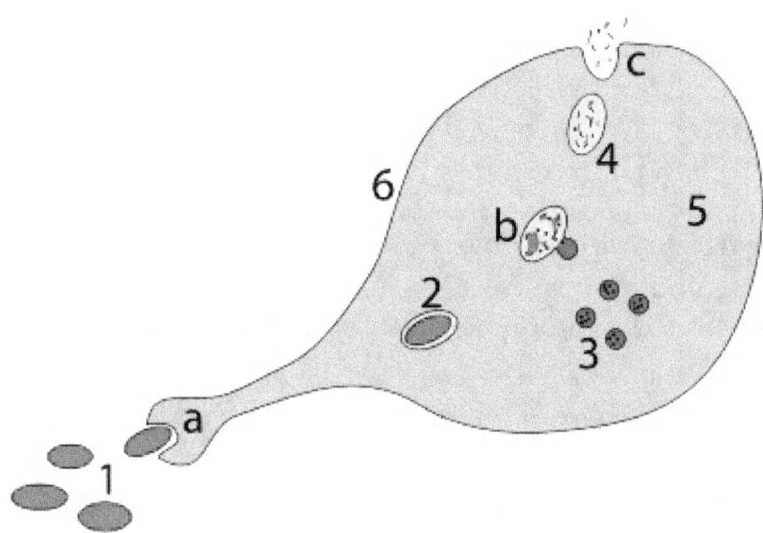

Steps of a macrophage ingesting a pathogen:

a. Ingestion through phagocytosis (large cell killers), a phagosome is formed

b. The fusion of lysosomes with the phagosome creates a phagolysosome; the pathogen is broken down by enzymes

c. Waste material is expelled or assimilated (the latter not pictured)

Phagocytosis means the engulfing and usually the destruction of particulate matter.

Lysosomes a saclike cellular organelle that contains various hydrolytic enzymes or a

tiny saclike part in a cell that contains enzymes which can break down materials (as

food particles and waste). Miriam Webster

Parts:1. Pathogens 2. Phagosome 3. Lysosomes 4. Waste Material 5. Cytoplasm 6.

Cell membrane Scanning electron micrograph of a phagocyte (yellow, right)

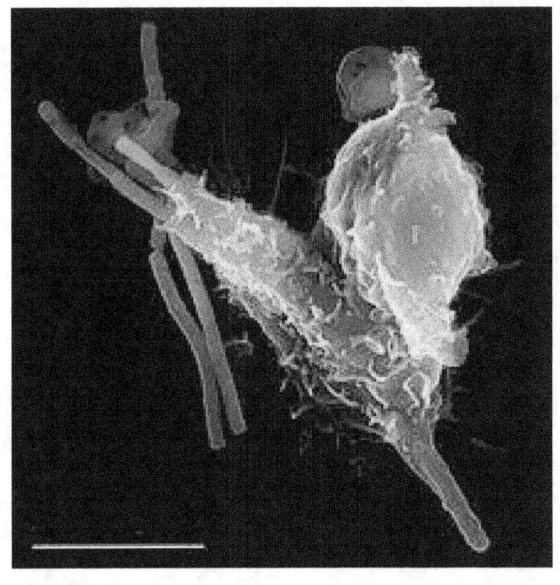

Phagocytosing anthrax bacilli (eating cells of

poison bacteria)

Scanning electron micrograph of a phagocyte (yellow, right) phagocytosing

anthrax bacilli (orange, left) Wikipedia phagocyte

The big eaters consume the anthrax and neutralize the disease proteins that they produce consumption of cells is what all this is saying. The body consumes and produces for energy and if the disease is more powerful from weakened immunity that with minerals is armed as the radiant power of the sun binds with mineral based proteins that in sufficient numbers neutralize diseases.

Phagocytes are cells that protect the body by ingesting (phagocytosing) harmful foreign particles, bacteria, and dead or dying cells. Their name comes from the Greek phagein, "to eat" or "devour", and "-cyte", the suffix in biology denoting "cell", from the Greek kutos, "hollow vessel". They are essential for fighting infections and for subsequent immunity. Phagocytes are important throughout the animal kingdom and are highly developed within vertebrates. One liter of human blood contains about six billion phagocytes.

Chemotherapy is a cytotoxic or cell killing therapy that is not specific to cancer but is chemical synthetization of known lethal venoms and chemicals that attack all cells causing immense damage to vital functions and has a deplorable survival rate of 2% when treated with the surgical, chemical toxic and manmade radiation that has legal backing with 600,000 deaths a year in 100-billion-dollar industry that will protect and vilify any challenge of truth. Studies of the power of natural healing are not sponsored and are recorded as unreliable. For example, the AMA ridiculed the Ayurveda, which is the medical mineral applications of India that dates 0ver 5000 years and is respected worldwide, for the use of arsenic a ubiquitous or widespread element in our environment and in miniscule amounts is healthy. At the same time, they use rat poison, mustard gas, spider venom and snake venom in cancer chemotherapy. Propaganda and misinformation is a media supported by advertising dollars lead you to pills and then lawsuits about bad drugs in a circus of money monkeys playing to an organ grinder (what they do) entertaining you as a medicine wagon tells you how great they are. They tell you that the cell killing or cytotoxic therapy has put the cancer in remission. This will then allow further treatment to keep it from coming back. Proper nutrition tips the scale for the elimination of the diseases ability to kill healthy cells. This is not remission but a program based on nature that stimulates healthy cells propagating by gaining control of your body in a survival of the fittest by cytotoxic advantage of disease cells that eliminate and aid in regeneration of tissue. When you take poison the disease forces are armed and immunity weakened and therefore the 2% survival rate and the additional problems of vital functions from the chemical bombardment of your cells that is masticated spontaneously by venoms and toxic compounds foreign to the immune system.

Mayo Clinic reports, "Antioxidant supplements, like vitamins C and E, might reduce the effectiveness of some types of cancer chemotherapy." So the cell killing poisons are attacked by vitamins to destroy the poisons. The power of nature to attack and destroy cancers is the best path and works if you allow natural holistic medicine.

They advertise with a list of disclaimers and do not tell of herbal curing even though all their medicine must match the natural receptors in our body. What they cannot do is absorb into the bloodstream and metabolic functions as herbs of organic source to organisms (us) do naturally and spillover to other receptors causing damage that can be fatal and at least drain energy which the antithesis of health and wellbeing. "Chemotherapy and radiation also reduce Nagalase levels. So does GcMAF" Dr. TJ Smith. So here is the choice. Your immunosuppressive in your body means that the immune system has been stopped and good forces have been disabled. Immune vitality comes from nutritional minerals that combine with the Sun's radiation that synthesize Vitamin D3 and combine with Amino Acids or protein to create GcMaf an enzyme that reduces disease without destroying other major functions of the body that can be lethal but rises the forces of immune vitality suppressing the Nagalase. To understand this further is that there is the flu season and that is when the sunlight is reduced and its radiation power to combine with protein for energy that suppresses virus is diminished as your energy reduces. So the sun's radiation is a natural power that reduces infection and helps with nutrition to gain and produce energy.

"Serum Vitamin D3-binding protein (Gc protein) is the precursor for the principal macrophage activating factor (MAF). The MAF precursor activity of serum Gc protein of breast cancer patients was lost or reduced because Gc protein was deglycosylated by serum alpha-N-acetylgalactosaminidase (Nagalase) secreted from cancerous cells. Patient serum Nagalase activity is proportional to Tumor burden. The deglycosylated Gc protein cannot be converted to MAF, resulting in no macrophage activation and immunosuppression. Stepwise incubation of purified Gc protein with immobilized beta-galactosidase and sialidase generated probably the most potent macrophage activating factor (termed GcMAF) ever discovered, which produces no adverse effect in humans. Macrophages treated in vitro with GcMAF (100 pg/ml) are highly tumoricidal to mammary adenocarcinomas. Efficacy of GcMAF for treatment of metastatic breast cancer was investigated with 16 nonanemic patients who received weekly administration of GcMAF (100 ng). As GcMAF therapy progresses, the MAF precursor activity of patient Gc protein increased with a concomitant decrease in serum Nagalase. Because of proportionality of serum Nagalase activity to tumor burden, the time course progress of GcMAF therapy was assessed by serum Nagalase activity as a prognostic index. These patients had the initial Nagalase activities ranging from 2.32 to 6.28 nmole/min/mg protein. After about 16-22 administrations (approximately 3.5-5 months) of GcMAF, these patients had insignificantly low serum enzyme levels equivalent to healthy control enzyme levels, ranging from 0.38 to 0.63 nmole/min/mg protein, indicating eradication of the tumors. This therapeutic

procedure resulted in no recurrence for more than 4 years." Publication: International journal

of cancer. Journal international du cancer Publication Date: 2008 Study Author(s): Yamamoto, Nobuto;Suyama,

Hirofumi;Yamamoto, Nobuyuki;Ushijima, Naofumi; Institution: Division of Cancer Immunology and Molecular

Biology, Socrates Institute for Therapeutic Immunology, Philadelphia, PA 19126-3305, USA.

nobutoyama@verizon.net

Energy is the basis of all health and herbal organic nutrients give energy in great ascorbic and efficient delivery to our metabolic function promoting health and arming immune system to combat disease.

"Approximately 25% of all prescription drugs currently in use are originally derived from plants. Furthermore, approximately 75% of new anticancer drugs marketed between 1981 and 2006 are derived from plant compounds. Despite this, only 10% of the estimated 250,000 species worldwide have been screened for any bioactivities. Plants produce a variety of biologically active compounds which exhibit an array of properties. The study of plant pharmacognosy could lead to the discovery of commercially and/or therapeutically useful phytochemicals possessing a diverse range of activities. As a result of its geographic isolation, Australia is home to a large variety of unique and distinct flora not found elsewhere in the world. Due to the harsh conditions seen in many parts of Australia, plants have developed unique survival methods specific to the environmental conditions they inhabit and may hold the key to the treatment of many diseases and medical conditions. Traditional Aboriginal knowledge of plants as therapeutics is disappearing as the Aboriginal culture merges

into main stream society and the passing of oral traditions between each generation diminishes. Given the diverse nature of the flora present and the diminishing traditional knowledge, Australian plants remain relatively unstudied and it is surprising that more research has not been done into their potential." Pharmacogn Rev. 2012 Jan-Jun; 6(11): 29–36.

The universe is equilibrium in time and space and within our body it plays out as alkaline and acid. If the acid is too strong then disease will surface. Cholesterol is called good and bad. When the body has not gotten enough minerals, vitamins and sunshine with nutrition Gc-maf is balanced. For the medical community to not follow this research means the healing process is blocked until the disease has killed cells and is growing. The lymphocytes that in the lymph glands fight infection with minerals that are bound to proteins to attack virus and cancer enzymes that are attacking their immune system to suppress healthy tissue. So nutrition and sunlight are a formidable force of the power of natural healing.

The Sun's radiation power is one of three main sources of health and depending on your pigmentation the need for it absorption for synthesizing to immune defenses varies. Along with this the environment gives you another powerful and natural element for health and vitality and this is Oxygen.

Chapter 3. Oxygen

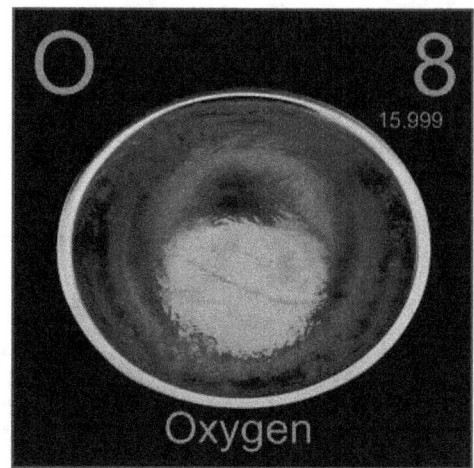

Oxygen is a gas that is 21% of the environment that is blue in color as a gas we breath and is hydrated in water that cleans the universe and helps detoxing our body as a cleaning action of a river Glycolysis (from glycose, an older term for glucose + -lysis degradation) is the metabolic pathway that converts glucose C6H12O6, into pyruvate, CH3COCOO− + H+. The free energy released in this process is used to form the high-energy compounds ATP (adenosine triphosphate) and NADH (reduced nicotinamide adenine dinucleotide)." This is the pathway for energy transfer within our cells and the process of synthesizing proteins by the bio-degradable nutrients that produce minerals for consumption and then produce molecular natural sugars that bind with radiated vitamins of metamorphosis that chemically synthesized proteins for immune defenses.

Doctor Wilson's explanation of deglycocosates is "deglycosylates (removes the sugars from) DBP. Deglycosylated DBP cannot be converted to GcMAF, thus it loses the GcMAF precursor activity, leading to immunosuppression." Diseases form proteins that are cytotoxic by neutralizing the glucose (ripened nutrition of sweetness of inner metabolic functions).

So Glycolsis is vital to immunity against disease and it is prebiotic phenomenon meaning that oxygen was the basis of the creation of life and a vital force or Pranayama

"Glycolysis is a determined sequence of ten enzyme-catalyzed reactions. The intermediates provide entry points to glycolysis. For example, most monosaccharides, such as fructose and galactose, can be converted to one of these intermediates. The intermediates may also be directly useful. For example, the intermediate dihydroxyacetone phosphate (DHAP) is a source of the glycerol that combines with fatty acids to form fat.

The Glycolysis is an oxygen independent metabolic pathway, meaning that it does not use molecular oxygen (i.e. atmospheric oxygen) for any of its reactions. However, the products of glycolysis (pyruvate and NADH + H+) are sometimes disposed of using atmospheric oxygen. When molecular oxygen is used in the disposal of the products of glycolysis the process is usually referred to as aerobic, whereas if the disposal uses no oxygen the process is said to be anaerobic. Thus, glycolysis occurs, with variations, in nearly all organisms, both aerobic and anaerobic. The wide occurrence of glycolysis indicates that it is one of the most ancient metabolic pathways. Indeed, the reactions that constitute glycolysis and its parallel pathway, the pentose phosphate pathway, occur metal-catalyzed under the oxygen-free conditions of the Archean oceans, also in the absence of enzymes. Glycolysis could thus have originated from chemical constraints of the prebiotic world. Keller; Ralser; Turchyn (Apr 2014). "Non-enzymatic glycolysis and pentose phosphate pathway-like reactions in a plausible Archean ocean". Mol Syst Biol. 10: 725. doi:10.1002/msb.20145228.PMID 24771084 *Glycolysis occurs in most organisms. The entire glycolysis pathway can be separated into two phases:*

ATP is consumed and produced to aid metabolic transfer of immune defense against immune suppression

ATP is the main source for the screening and allowing communication for energy transfer in molecular connections. If this enzyme is disabled, then cells are invaded. This same ATP is found in plants and allows the storage of radiant energy for food production.

As you can see the basis of life is the Sun and Oxygen combining to create an atmosphere for the survival of biotic and this primal force is the basis of immune power of nature to survive the attack of disease this is the survival of the fittest. This purity of energy can heal and survive and we see this in the world of both plant and animal.

The plants provide oxygen that we breathe that helps create energy. The minerals drawn from the ground by the radiant energy of the sun matching organic receptors of our body in a chemical electrical universe synthesizing into energy in a metamorphic regeneration of our body and mind. We have been in this relationship for all time. They want to create body parts using supercell technology and we have the power from birth when at conception the supercell began constructing our body.

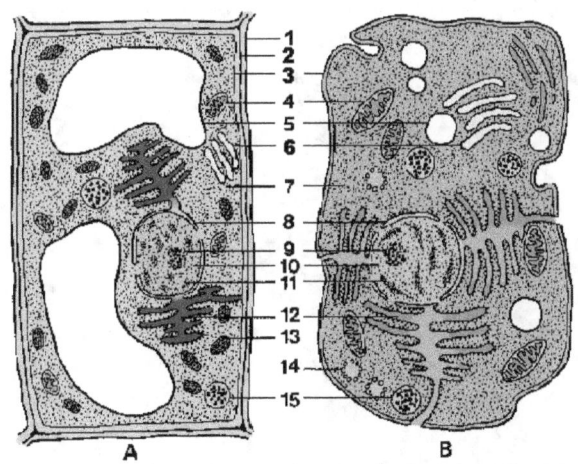

Cell 4 (schematic): A plant, B animal; 1 cell wall, 2 middle lamella, 3 plasma membrane, 4 mitochondrion, 5 vacuole, 6 Golgi apparatus, 7 cytoplasm, 8 nuclear membrane, 9 nucleolus, 10 nucleus, 11 chromatin, 12 endoplasmic reticulum with associated ribosomes, 13 chloroplast, 14 centriole, 15 lysosome. Merriam Webster

The cell structure of plant and animal have the same biology for cell growth and energy manipulation

"Photosynthesis

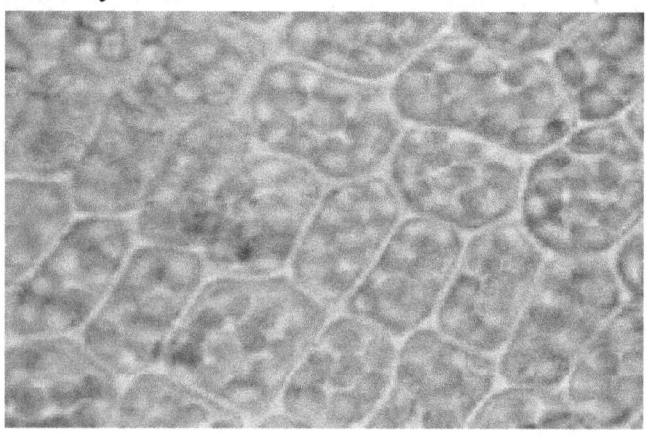

The process by which some, photosynthetic, organisms use the energy of sunlight to produce sugars.

All organisms need energy, food, to survive, but only plants, algae, and some bacteria are able to produce it themselves. They use the Sun's energy to make glucose (a carbohydrate) from water (H_2O) and carbon dioxide (CO_2). The process also produces the oxygen humans and other organisms breathe. $6H_2O + 6CO_2 \rightarrow C_6H_{12}O_6 + 6O$ Plants catch the energy of sunlight in a pigment in their leaves, chlorophyll, which makes them green.

Like other organisms, plants will use some of the glucose themselves through respiration. But a large part of the energy trapped by photosynthetic organisms is eventually transferred to other organisms, herbivores, which eat plants and algae.

Therefore, almost all living organisms directly or indirectly depend on photosynthesis. Animals, which cannot photosynthesize themselves, depend on photosynthetic organisms for food. Through photosynthesis, CO_2 is removed from the atmosphere and built into organic matter, for example trees. When trees die and decomposes the carbon is eventually released back into the atmosphere. This is a natural part of the carbon cycle.

If the balance between photosynthesis and respiration is changed it could influence global warming. Destruction of forests would increase the content of CO_2 in the atmosphere. On the other hand, increased photosynthesis, i.e. more plants, would help reduce the amount of CO_2 in the atmosphere." http://climap.net/photosynthesis Minerals that are in plants I refer to as Soft Metals that are metabolized for energy to regenerate our body. They are found for consumption in greatest and purest in organic food and therefore have an immense effect upon immune defenses when disease is attacking your body reducing energy.

Chapter 4. Stem Cells & Embryogenesis

The power of nature is omnipotent and it is a sacred gift with the equal or greater than any medicine. We are born vegetarians through which the vast construction of trillions of connections by stem cells from a DNA blueprint built our bodies with an immune system against all odds to be born. The weakening of this system in a highly toxic environment has caused an alarming rate of cancer and autistic levels. Maintenance of the stem cells will allow this powerful natural immunity to flourish. The key is to extend the mineral based food that was the yoke of nutrition for our immune system. Let's take a look at the scientific information and where the instruments play in octaves to regenerate daily. The research is intense to discover how the stem cells work. They already have isolated a Super Cell that is the conductor of a symphony. By doing this they have constructed a heart but without life or metabolic function. If they can do this, then you can do it! In a lab they grew a heart. They used minerals to achieve this. There is no other way. All medicine is developed by matching the natural receptors in the body. For example, serotonin is transmitted from the Pineal Gland between the two hemispheres of the brain and this is a primal force from inception. Anxiety pills match up with these receptors so the pill is some form of natural elements. So the herbalists and naturalists have the necessary herbs to replicate any pill but with a major difference. Nature metabolizes the input to your body specifically to the receptors without additional direct contact to receptors that are not a match. Pills go to many receptors that are called side effects but are a direct assault upon the body. Therefore, the disclaimers of many possible diseases are listed. The research upon natural herbs is only scratching the surface. There are thousands of natural occurring plants have yet to reveal to us. Nutrition is consumption of the rainbow of colored plants for the production of energy that heals and the purest form of this can heal all diseases.

Neural stem cells or the NCS are self-renewing, multipotent cells that generate the main phenotype of the CNS or central nervous system. Stem cells differentiate into multiple cell types with exogenous stimuli from minerals and environment or foods that are eaten with mineral and vitamin strength. They undergo cell division asymmetrically into two daughter cells. NCS differentiate primarily into neurons, astrocytes.

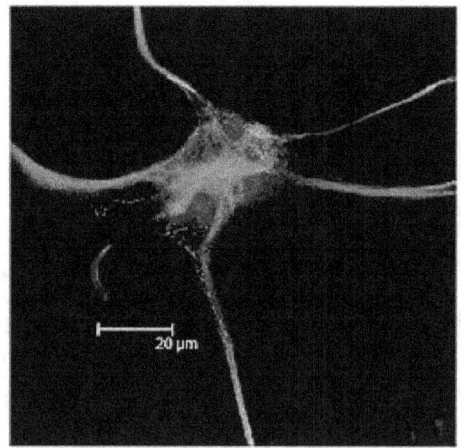

Astrocytes (Astro from Greek astron = star and cyte from Greek "kyttaron" = cell), also known collectively as astroglia, are characteristic star-shaped glial cells in the brain and spinal cord. Glia cells aid the transmission and glia means glue in Greek and they support neurotransmitters and protect the system. The proportion of astrocytes in the brain is not well defined. Depending on the counting technique used, studies have found that the astrocyte proportion varies by region and ranges from 20% to 40% of all glia. They perform many functions, including biochemical support of endothelial cells that form the blood–brain barrier, provision of nutrients to the nervous tissue, maintenance of extracellular ion balance, and a role in the repair and scarring process of the brain and spinal cord following traumatic injuries.

"Research since the mid-1990s has shown that astrocytes propagate intercellular Ca2+ waves over long distances in response to stimulation, and, similar to neurons, release transmitters (called gliotransmitters) in a Ca2+-dependent manner. Data suggest that astrocytes also signal to neurons through Ca2+-dependent release of glutamate. Such discoveries have made astrocytes an important area of research within the field of neuroscience." Wikipedia Stem Cells

We are chemically synthesized and we metabolize energy with nutrients that form light in an illusion of colors that race through the universe. Our link with nature is shown in the plants embryogenesis and the ripening of the fruits and vegetables that are

nutrition for us and how we ripen internally to molecular sugars that are proteins of immune strength when the sun's radiation binds with this as it does in plants.

Plants are fertilized and sprout and take root to extract nutrients and spread foliage to capture sunlight and the radiant energy for photosynthesis. We capture sunlight and convert it into vitamins feeding our body with nutrition. We are mobile and communicate and plants are stationary and communicate with pollen and odors to attract bees to reproduce. Embryogenesis occurs naturally as a result of sexual fertilization and the formation of the zygotic embryos. The embryo along with other cells from the mother plant develops into the seed or the next generation, which, after germination, grows into a new plant.

Embryogenesis may be divided up into two phases, the first involves morphogenetic events which form the basic cellular pattern for the development of the shoot-root body and the primary tissue layers; it also programs the regions of meristematic tissue formation. The second phase, or postembryonic development, involves the maturation of cells, which involves cell growth and the storage of macromolecules (such as oils, starches and proteins) required as a 'food and energy supply' during germination and seedling growth. Embryogenesis involves cell growth and division, cell differentiation and programmed cellular death. The zygotic embryo is formed following double fertilization of the ovule, giving rise to two distinct structures: the plant embryo and the endosperm which together go on to develop into a seed. Seeds may also develop without fertilization, which is referred to as apomixes. Plant cells can also be induced to form embryos in plant tissue culture; such embryos are called somatic embryos and can be used to generate new plants from single cells.

"Following fertilization, the zygote undergoes an asymmetrical cell division that gives rise to a small apical cell, which becomes the embryo and a large basal cell (called the suspensor), which functions to provide nutrients from the endosperm to the growing embryo. From the eight cell stage (octant stage) onwards, the zygotic embryo shows clear embryo patterning, which forms the main axis of polarity, and the linear formation of future structures. These structures include the shoot meristem, cotyledons, hypocotyl, and the root and root meristem: they arise from specific groups of cells as the young embryo divides and their formation has been shown to be position-dependent". ZMBP Embryo Patterning

The wild tobacco plant when a caterpillar feeds upon it excretes an odor that attracts a predator that eats caterpillars. We are like trees that spread their leaves to capture radiation from the sun and chemically synthesize with nutrition from the ground with this radiation to grow food. We with these minerals feed the Super Cell that feeds the stem cells for regeneration of tissue with this captured radiant food. When we are first conceived energy is present and we form into our body and this is the genesis of life with nature as the power.

Stem cells are very powerful and women have reproductive stem cells for birth. This is a primal force of nature and is kindled for reproduction and is the basic core of energy manipulation of the Chakras Which ancient India identified as Energy Centers. The same energy is in the male or Shiva and Shakti in female. What is amazing is the ancient understanding and cultivation of this power.

Also the understanding of metabolic power by consuming plants that are a primary source of primal forces of food. animal food is a second hand basis of mineral consumption but the fish have purer nutrition due to the sea or water connection to nutrients. Plants have a pure chemical synthesized nutrition brought through stems and synthesized with radiation utilizing ATP enzyme to store energy as it does in us.

"Embryogenesis is the process by which the embryo forms and develops. In mammals, the term refers chiefly to early stages of prenatal development, whereas the terms fetus and fetal development describe later stages.

"Embryogenesis starts with the fertilization of the egg cell (ovum) by a sperm cell, (spermatozoon). Once fertilized, the ovum is referred to as a zygote, a single diploid cell. The zygote undergoes mitotic divisions with no significant growth (a process

known as cleavage) and cellular differentiation, leading to development of a multicellular embryo.

Embryogenesis occurs in both animal and plant development, this article addresses the common features among different animals, with some emphasis on the embryonic development of vertebrates and mammals."

Here we can see clearly that plants and animals share unique growth patterns and this is why the organic food radiated by the sun match the production through consumption of our organic chemical electrical synthesis that produces polymers and steroids from the mineral harvest of nutrition that was the genesis at our conception.

Polarity in embryogenesis is the early development of the body and during this period our body is mapped out by the stem cell branching out to build our body and mind. The body is divided into two hemispheres called the animal pole and the vegetal pole. The animal pole is rapidly growing and in natures perfect balance the vegetal pole is slow and supplies the nutrition for early metabolism through the stems cells.

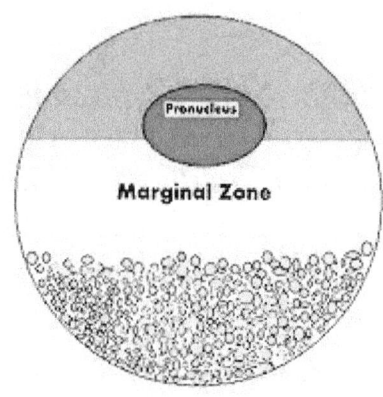

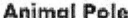

In developmental biology, an embryo is divided into two hemispheres: the animal pole and the vegetal pole within a blastula.

The animal pole consists of small cells that divide rapidly, in contrast with the vegetal pole below it. The animal pole draws its name from its liveliness relative to the slowly developing vegetal pole. In some cases, the animal pole is thought to differentiate into the later embryo itself, forming the three primary germ layers and participating in gastrulation. Sperm enters the egg at the animal pole.

The vegetal pole contains large yolky cells that divide very slowly, in contrast with the animal pole above it. The vegetal pole draws its name from its inactivity relative to the lively animal pole. In some cases, the vegetal pole is thought to differentiate into the extraembryonic membranes that protect and nourish the developing embryo, such as the placenta in mammals and the chorion in birds." wikipedia.org/wiki/Polarity_in_embryogenesis

The plants have ATP that helps the storage of radiant energy for photosynthesis. This enzyme plays a significant role in neurotransmitter connections in our body by limiting permeability to the cells in a balance of natural energy to aid in barriers to cellular integrity for efficient functions.

When a plant breaks down with oxygen it shoots out new growth to start new life like in a potato. Trees drop seeds on the forest floor where there is humus that helps oxygenate the seedlings for new growth. Within us we are in a constant state of metamorphosis from the beginning of our lives at the moment of fertilization our body stems out to create our phenotype and functions that make us healthy and to have wellbeing. We soak in the sun to chemically synthesize radiant energy into energy for health. When you begin to understand that we are part of nature and that trillions of receptors respond to natural stimulation from plants that have regenerated to form soft metals of iron, magnesium and others to fuel metabolic functions that create energy for life you will feel healthy and have wellbeing. The only way to feel and understand this ultimate power is to practice the sun exposure, breath to the max and eat nutritious so the elements can consume and produce the metabolic pathway for stunning results. Short of this is short of metabolic pathways being constructed to its maximum development. If you are on this journey, you stop before the destination. The natural path is slower than pills or immediate gratification. One must strive to soak in the sun's radiation over time and to expand respiration for circulation and eat nutritious is a journey that will lead you to a treasure of life. Nature is nurturing and as you have seen the start of our lives in the embryogenesis this pattern of nurturing is slow as we grow rapidly from the nurturing. When you suffer from a virus minerals and vitamins with the radiant sunlight will rid the body of symptoms by destroying the virus and in a few gays the sickness will go away completely not lingering on with coughing as pills leave you because they relieve symptoms and only give you time to build up immunity whereas immunity is minerals and vitamins.

During the embryo development the feeding is established to provide nutrition for the metabolic functions growing the body from a blueprint using nutrition of minerals to aid the stem cells in growth. Here the gastro intestinal function develops for consumption to grow for nutrition is a most important step and the healing power

 "Gastrulation is a phase early in the embryonic development of most animals, during which the single-layered blastula is reorganized into a trilaminar ("three-layered") structure known as the gastrula. These three germ layers are known as the ectoderm, mesoderm, and endoderm.

Gastrulation takes place after cleavage and the formation of the blastula. Gastrulation is followed by organogenesis, when individual organs develop within the newly formed germ layers. Each layer gives rise to specific tissues and organs in the developing embryo. The ectoderm gives rise to epidermis, and to the neural crest and other tissues *that will later form the nervous system. The mesoderm is found between the ectoderm and the endoderm and gives rise to somites, which form muscle; the cartilage of the ribs and vertebrae; the dermis, the notochord, blood and blood vessels ,bone, and connective tissue. The endoderm gives rise to the epithelium of the digestive system and respiratory system, and organs associated with the <u>digestive system</u>, such as the liver and pancreas. Following gastrulation, cells in the body are either organized into sheets of connected cells (as in epithelia), or as a mesh of isolated cells.*

The molecular mechanism and timing of gastrulation is different in different organisms. However, some common features of gastrulation across triploblastic organisms include: (1) A change in the topological structure of the embryo, from a simply connected surface (sphere-like), to a non-simply connected surface (torus-like); (2) the differentiation of cells into one of three types (endodermal, mesodermal, and ectodermal); and (3) the digestive function of a large number of endodermal cells. wikipedia.org/wiki/Gastrulation

Lewis Wolpert, *pioneering developmental biologist in the field, has been credited for noting that "It is not birth, marriage, or death, but gastrulation, which is truly the most important time in your life."* wikipedia.org/wiki/Lewis_Wolpert

As you can see the early development of the immune system in the gastrointestinal system is to nourish and develop filtering organs as the liver and connective tissues with respiration for oxygen cleaning vessels.

When ancient civilizations were close to nature they realized the union with nature much more clearly and also faced hardships that we do not in our modern culture. This is to our detriment physically and mentally. This is witnessed by the diseases and drug usage to overcome the toxins in our physical and mental environment. The process of the plant world is like ours and the link with nature is paramount for physical and mental wellbeing.

"Plant embryogenesis is the process that produces a plant embryo from a fertilized ovule by asymmetric cell division and the differentiation of undifferentiated cells into tissues and organs. It occurs during seed development, when the single-celled zygote undergoes a programmed pattern of cell division resulting in a mature embryo. A similar process continues during the plant's life within the meristems of the stems and roots

Embryogenesis occurs naturally as a result of sexual fertilization and the formation of the zygotic embryos. The embryo along with other cells from the mother plant develops into the seed or the next generation, which, after germination, grows into a new plant.

Embryogenesis may be divided up into two phases, the first involves morphogenetic events which form the basic cellular pattern for the development of the shoot-root body and the primary tissue layers; it also programs the regions of meristematic tissue formation. The second phase, or postembryonic development, involves the maturation of cells, which involves cell growth and the storage of macromolecules (such as oils, starches and proteins) required as a 'food and energy supply' during germination and seedling growth. Embryogenesis involves cell growth and division, cell differentiation and programmed cellular death. The zygotic embryo is formed following double fertilization of the ovule, giving rise to two distinct structures: the plant embryo and the endosperm which together go on to develop into a seed. Seeds may also develop without fertilization, which is referred to as apomixes. Plant cells can also be induced to form embryos in plant tissue culture; such embryos are called somatic embryos and can be used to generate new plants from single cells.

Following fertilization, the zygote undergoes an asymmetrical cell division that gives rise to a small apical cell, which becomes the embryo and a large basal cell (called the suspensor), which functions to provide nutrients from the endosperm to the growing embryo. From the eight cell stage (octant stage) onwards, the zygotic embryo shows clear embryo patterning, which forms the main axis of polarity, and the linear formation of future structures. These structures include the shoot meristem, cotyledons, hypocotyl, and the root and root meristem: they arise from specific groups of cells as the young embryo divides and their formation has been shown to be position-dependent." wikipedia.org/wiki/Plant embryogenesis

When you look at the ancient Chakras or Energy Centers there are 7 main ones that begin in the gastrointestinal tract and move ascending to the crown of the head enhancing the Aura Chakra light emission. Our body establishes this connection from conception with the mineral based nourishment for maximum growth. this growth mirrors the plant world and we both use respiration to remove toxins.

"The process by which some photosynthetic organisms use the energy of sunlight to produce sugars. All organisms need energy, food, to survive, but only plants, algae, and some bacteria are able to produce it themselves. They use the Sun's energy to make glucose (a carbohydrate) from water (H_2O) and carbon dioxide (CO_2). The process also produces the oxygen humans and other organisms breathe.

Plants catch the energy of sunlight in a pigment in their leaves, chlorophyll, which makes them green.

Like other organisms, plants will use some of the glucose themselves through respiration. But a large part of the energy trapped by photosynthetic organisms is eventually transferred to other organisms, herbivores, which eat plants and algae.

Therefore, almost all living organisms directly or indirectly depend on photosynthesis.

Animals, which cannot photosynthesize themselves, depend on photosynthetic

organisms for food.

Through photosynthesis, CO_2 is removed from the atmosphere and built into organic

matter, for example trees. When trees die and decomposes the carbon is eventually

released back into the atmosphere. This is a natural part of the carbon cycle.

If the balance between photosynthesis and respiration is changed it could influence

global warming. Destruction of forests would increase the content of CO_2 in the

atmosphere. On the other hand, increased photosynthesis, i.e. more plants, would help

reduce the amount of CO_2 in the atmosphere." http://climap.net/photosynthesis

The body immune system defense and attack is demonstrated in Antioxidants and

shows the accepted ability because of market profit. " An antioxidant is a molecule

that inhibits the oxidation of other molecules. Oxidation is a chemical reaction

involving the loss of electrons or an increase in oxidation state. Oxidation reactions

can produce free radicals. In turn, these radicals can start chain reactions. When the

chain reaction occurs in a cell, it can cause damage or death to the cell. Antioxidants

terminate these chain reactions by removing free radical intermediates, and inhibit

other oxidation reactions. They do this by being oxidized themselves, so antioxidants

are often reducing agents such as thiols, ascorbic acid (vitamin C), or polyphenols." [Sies]

H (Mar 1997). "Oxidative stress: oxidants and antioxidants". Experimental Physiology 82 (2): 291–5. doi:10.1113/exp

physiol.1997.sp004024.PMID 9129943.

As you see this is a perfect example of how fruits and vegetables or nutrition defend the body by removing free radicals with vitamin C through a metamorphosis of nutrients that energize on the molecular level where toxins need to be removed.

The respiration of the plants and animals is the creation of energy by the breakdown of matter through a constant metamorphosis. Interference from variables in this balanced continuum causes an adjustment on the micro and macro scale of nature. The process of yoga includes breath control or the vital force of Pranayama enhancing this energy. The three pillars of Nature are the Sun, Oxygen and Nutrition that the earth sky and space combine for energy and vitality.

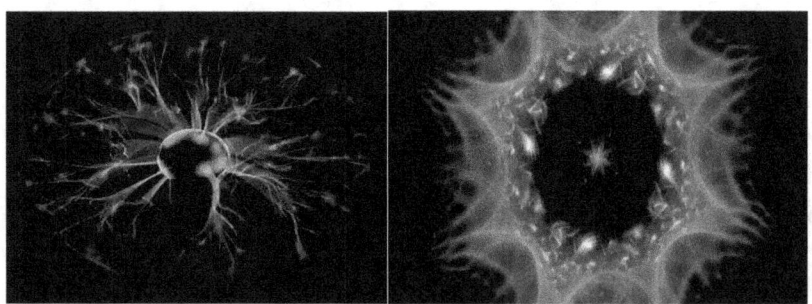

The first picture is a plasma globe. Plasma fuels the Aurora Borealis and the adjacent picture is Super Nova in the heavens. The universe out there is in you including plasma which is primordial solution of our atomic cells stemming outward to generate and regenerate and with nutrients the body is exalted as a temple in purity free of disease.

Chapter 5 Sugar The Good, Bad and Ugly

Sugar is in many forms and is a very, very important aid to the body for cognitive skills and immunity. Through the process of consuming minerals and vitamins the body produces amino acids that are proteins. These are a ripening as is in nature. Take an apple tree for example. It ripens with photosynthesis from solar energy by drawing minerals from the earth and when it is sweet and savory it is at its height of nutrition and drops this to the earth to replenish minerals and vitamins for regeneration of plants. Manipulations of this is bad that can turn ugly.

We subject our children to an all-out attack of bad sugar in doses that make them hyper active and cause brain damage. When you see a child acting this out think about what is happening to the brain. Recently I saw a child in a grocery isle with sugar laden cereals with cartoon characters in every combination of primary colors and on the opposite side of the isle was candy in every attempt to mesmerize the child to rot his teeth, body and mind.

Within our body as the vitamins and minerals become ripened they have travelled through the many functions of the immune system such as liver and kidneys to metamorphose into powerful proteins that bind with solar energy that has travelled for 7 days to create a compound that arms the Lymph glands that send out Lymphocytes. These are infused into the bloodstream as Big Eaters or Macro Phages that are 5 billion strong in a well fed with nutrition versus toxins that fight the production of dead cell proteins that are powerful disease. This is the battle or the survival of the fittest. When the dead cells from tobacco, alcohol, preservatives and pesticides create a cocktail that deadens cells the dead cell produce Nagalase a protein that is the first stage of disease. In order for the disease to progress it must destroy the Big Eaters and granulated sugar or modified sugar is what powers the toxic proteins.

The Nagalase wants to survive and with natural sugar from minerals we can destroy the precursor of disease. Understand that the body has a balance and when we abuse it with chemicals the diseases surface in the bloodstream first and attack the weak points of the body. Strength from immunity built upon minerals, vitamins and solar power can destroy in the bloodstream the disease proteins that are trying to attack our weak points. So the best proteins are synthesized in our chemical electrical system that are amino acid sugars and granulated manipulated sugar arms the disease that takes over the bloodstream if not destroyed by natural process. This is the basis of survival of the fittest.

Because sugar for negative and positive forces of immunity is equally important one should be vigilant about what rots the teeth and the body this is discussed further to warn you of how it is a culprit.

First of all, they say it is an appetite suppressor and you won't eat food. They are right sugar kills your appetite but what it does is mess with your immune metabolic system that with minerals from fruits and vegetables produce sugars that are natural energy for immune system. When you consume food the body rewards you with a full feeling and releases serotonin that satisfies. This is a primal force that we get from hunting and eating for energy. The pseudo sugars trick the mind that you have eaten. However, as the man made sugars wear off you are feeling you have eaten nothing at all and your energy is hallow feeling, which is the case. The energy that is given from these sugars are negative forces in the body. The proteins from dead cells rotting thrive on this and studies, though suppressed, show the danger of High Fructose Corn Syrup and the power of natural sugar that arms the immunity, as these following articles explain.

When a tree produces fruits there is a mature time when the nutrition is at its peak from sweetening process of natural sugars. Within our body these minerals sweeten in a fermentation that produces protein amino acids that are natural sugars from the source of radiated fruits and plants to the radiated fruits of our body that create energy by breaking down with respiration utilizing oxygen. This is energy.

"The D-isomer (D-glucose) occurs widely in nature, but the L-isomer (L-glucose) does not. Glucose is made during photosynthesis from water and carbon dioxide, using

energy from sunlight. The reverse of the photosynthesis reaction, which releases this energy, is a very important source of power for cellular respiration. Glucose is stored as a polymer, in plants as starch and in animals as glycogen.

Glucose is a ubiquitous fuel in biology. It is used as an energy source in most organisms, from bacteria to humans, through either aerobic respiration, anaerobic respiration, or fermentation. Glucose is the human body's key source of energy, through aerobic respiration, providing about 3.75 kilocalories (16 kilojoules) of food energy per gram. Breakdown of carbohydrates (e.g. starch) yields mono- and disaccharides, most of which is glucose. Through glycolysis and later in the reactions of the citric acid cycle and oxidative phosphorylation, glucose is oxidized to eventually form CO_2 and water, yielding energy mostly in the form of ATP. The insulin reaction, and other mechanisms, regulate the concentration of glucose in the blood.

Glucose supplies almost all the energy for the brain, so its availability influences psychological processes. When glucose is low, psychological processes requiring mental effort (e.g., self-control, effortful decision-making) are impair In the U.S., HFCS is among the sweeteners that mostly replaced sucrose (table sugar) in the food industry.[9] Factors include production quotas of domestic sugar, import tariff on foreign sugar, and subsidies of U.S. corn, raising the price of sucrose and lowering that of HFCS, making it cheapest for many sweetener applications. The relative sweetness of HFCS 55, used most commonly in soft drinks, is comparable to sucrose.

Because of its superficially similar sugar profile and lower price, HFCS has been used illegally to "stretch" honey. Assays to detect adulteration with HFCA use differential scanning calorimetry and other advanced testing methods.

Sugars became a health concern among the American public in the early 1970s with the publication of John Yudkin's book, Pure, White and Deadly, which claimed that simple sugars, an increasingly large part of the Western diet, were dangerous: In the 1980s and 1990s Gerald Reaven and Sheldon Reiser of the USDA published papers discussing the dangers of dietary fructose from consumption of sucrose and of HFCS, especially with regard to heart disease, diabetes, and obesity. These concerns came to the public's attention through media attention to a 2004 commentary in The American Journal of Clinical Nutrition that suggested that the altered metabolism of fructose when compared to glucose may be a factor in increasing obesity rates since, as compared to glucose, fructose may be more readily converted to fat and the sugar causes less of a rise in insulin and leptin, both of which increase feelings of satiety. Fructose, in contrast to glucose, was shown to potently stimulate lipogenesis (creation of fatty acids, for conversion to fat). In subsequent interviews, two of the study's authors stated the article was distorted to place emphasis solely on HFCS when the actual issue was the overconsumption of any type of sugar. While fructose absorption and modification by the intestines and liver does differ from glucose initially, the majority of the fructose molecules are converted to glucose or metabolized into byproducts identical to those produced by glucose metabolism. Consumption of moderate amounts of fructose has also been linked to positive outcomes, including reducing appetite if consumed before a meal, lower blood sugar increases compared to glucose, and (again compared to glucose) delaying exhaustion if consumed during exercise.

In 2007 an expert panel assembled by the University of Maryland's Center for Food, Nutrition and Agriculture Policy reviewed the links between HFCS and obesity and concluded there was no ecological validity in the association between rising body mass indexes (a measure of obesity) and the consumption of HFCS. The panel stated that since the ratio of fructose to glucose had not changed substantially in the United States since the 1960s when HFCS was introduced, the changes in obesity rates were probably not due to HFCS specifically but rather a greater consumption of calories overall, and recommended further research on the topic. In 2009 the American Medical Association published a review article on HFCS and concluded that based on the science available at the time it appeared unlikely that HFCS contributed more to obesity or other health conditions than sucrose, and there was insufficient evidence to suggest warning about or restricting use of HFCS or other fructose-containing sweeteners in foods. The review did report that studies found direct associations between high intakes of fructose and adverse health outcomes, including obesity and the metabolic syndrome.

Epidemiological research has suggested that the increase in metabolic disorders like obesity and non-alcoholic fatty liver disease, is linked to increased consumption of sugars and/or calories in general, and not due to any special effect of HFCS. A 2012 review found that fructose did not appear to cause weight gain when it replaced other carbohydrates in diets with similar calories. High fructose consumption has been linked to high levels of uric acid in the blood, though this is only thought to be a concern for patients with gout. [4]

Numerous agencies in the United States recommend reducing the consumption of all sugars, including HFCS, without singling it out as presenting extra concerns. The Mayo Clinic cites the American Heart Association's recommendation that women limit the added sugar in their diet to 100 calories a day (~6 teaspoons) and that men limit it to 150 calories a day (~9 teaspoons), noting that there is not enough evidence to support HFCS having more adverse health effects than excess consumption of any other type of sugar.[44][45] The United States departments of Agriculture and Health and Human Services recommendations for a healthy diet state that consumption of all types of added sugars be reduced.

People with fructose malabsorption should avoid foods containing HFCS.

One implication of the finding that carbohydrate restriction in obese patients causes them to lose weight is that excessive carbohydrate consumption is likely to be a cause of obesity in the first place. An obvious possible culprit is sugar, which provides calories but no nutrients whatever. Given the dramatic increase in sugar consumption during the first half of the century, Yudkin started to suspect that excessive sugar in the diet might contribute not only to obesity but also to coronary heart disease. Studying historical data from many different countries, he found that increasing prosperity leads to an increase in sugar consumption, particularly in manufactured foods, and also that the ready availability of sugar-containing manufactured foods even in the poorer countries may lead to their being bought in preference to more nutritious food. In 1964 he wrote 'In the wealthier countries, there is evidence that sugar and sugar-containing foods contribute to several diseases, including obesity, dental caries, diabetes mellitus and myocardial infarction [heart attack]'.

Investigating whether any link between sugar consumption and disease could be shown in individual patients, he and his associates in the Department of Nutrition found that patients with atherosclerotic disease (a frequent precursor of coronary heart disease) consumed significantly more sucrose than control patients.] An obstacle to the acceptance of these ideas was the belief at the time that sugar and starch were metabolized in the same way, so that one would expect no difference in their effects. Yudkin and his associates, however, fed both experimental animals and human volunteers with differing quantities of sugar and starch, and found major differences between the two carbohydrates in their metabolic effects. As early as 1967 Yudkin suggested that the excessive consumption of sugar might result in a disturbance in the secretion of insulin, and that this in turn might contribute to atherosclerosis and diabetes". Wikipedia HFCS

So the controversy goes on and those that deny it are protecting the investment of billions that have a sweet tooth they want to addict the population too whether or not it has a plethora of diseases it helps start and fuel. Watch the sugar in grams and reduce what you and your family ingests of this and the quality of energy will boost your metabolic pathways.

The shelves are filled with this pseudo energy drinks. Some use 6000 times the daily requirement of protein B12. This is overload to such an extent the body will have serious dependency issues and long term effects that are on the negative side of immunity. The drinks are filled with HFCS and other chemicals that aid in disease fuel. The food from one end of the grocery store to the other are listed with a lot of sugar. 4 grams of sugar is approximately one tsp of sugar. Many foods have 4 or more tsp of sugar and our daily intake is staggering especially if it is the bad sugar.

Energy is what we consume and produce and bad sugars are consumed and produce disease by giving them energy to attack the body, a fuel for disease.

When advertising and support for sugar laden health products are put on the market it can be aiding the negative sugar effect on the body like Ensure. Touted as a major nutrition aid and is given to cancer patients where chemo therapy of poison is daunting their appetite. This drink has 4-6 tsp of sugar per bottle and a trusted source of Natural News and the Health Ranger Mike Adams tested the Ensure ingredients and found, "Mike Adams, Editor of NaturalNews.com, extols in Ensure is Primarily Sugar Water, Marketed with Misleading Statements that Deceive Consumers:

"... the top two ingredients in Ensure are almost identical to the top two ingredients in soft drinks! ... the top four ingredients (are): water, sugar, corn syrup and maltodextrin. That's basically three sweeteners and water. So if you were trying to be funny, you could call this product 'sugar-sugar-sugar-water,' because that is primarily what it's made of, according to the ingredients label... So essentially, what

you have here with Ensure, is a predominantly sugar-water product that has been fortified with a few vitamins and minerals.

"The phrase, 'Complete, balanced, nutrition,' in my personal opinion, is an outright lie. This product has nothing resembling complete, balanced nutrition...

"This is one of a line of products that includes items like Slim fast and other meal replacement products that are primarily nothing but sugar-water and yet are promoted as healthy products that either provide optimum nutrition or promote weight loss...

"Products like Ensure or Slim Fast seem to imply that they are serious products for optimum nutrition, but in fact, an honest analysis of these products reveals that they offer extremely poor nutrition and they probably do far more harm than good to people who choose to consume them on a regular basis, as any good nutritionist will tell you."

Yes, you are not hungry because they have used sugar to trick the body into signaling being full and aiding the disease proteins gain energy.

Chapter 6.   Breath of Life

Page 252 of Vendata Bulletin: "Control of breath through science of breath can Command the body to do anything. The power of self-control is bound to come to one Who has learnt the control of breath or one who has faithfully practiced the breathing?

Exercises as given by the Swamis from India. The utility of this wonderful science is proved by medical practitioners, mental scientists, and by those who teach physical Culture or voice culture. Again, when this breath is brought under control it brings peace of mind. When the mind is directed towards the Supreme Ideal, you will obtain spiritual enlightenment, in which you will discover the past and future of your soul-life. Thus Raja Yoga when properly applied to our daily lives will make us strong logical."

Pranayama is not only freshness for our body but is the cleansing agent of the universe. There are many instances that we use oxygen to clean. When we wash anything we use water which is hydrated oxygen. There are also cleaning agents and medicinal applications such as Oxyclean and Hydrogen Peroxide. This follows suit with the power of cleansing in the universe of respiration and the ever present from the beginning of time the air we breathe. The earth uses rain and thunderstorms with lightning from the sky and earth to cleanse itself. When things become imbalanced typhoons and tsunamis form. When you get sick your body defends by washing out the toxins and raising temperature to increase metabolic chemical synthesis and need replenished minerals and vitamins from an organic source for an organism that is invaded by disease. The body with its immune system has a precision orchestrated disease attack mechanism and this is amino acids that are proteins bind with Vitamin D chemically creating an attack upon all diseases. Therefore, the sun's radiation increasing Vitamin D aids our nutrients with the most powerful immunity that bombards disease at the source of infection where the toxic disease is attacking our body. Pills attack the entire body leading to a euphemism of side effects that is a vast difference of pills that are not metabolic efficient in the matrix of connections that are in the trillions. Oncologist use radiation machines that are a poor substitute of the Sun's power to develop pigmentation of our skin and supply Vitamin D to bind with proteins to attack disease in a metabolic direct energy healing process. Add to this the oxygen the toxins are removed by respiration and bodily functions ridding your body of disease.

Water with oxygen aid in the washing out of the toxins and organic food metabolizes immune defense system. The circulatory system is enhanced as the breath control is increased with manipulation making your delivery of immune system better. Therefore; an increased circulatory and respiratory will clean out toxins with increased oxygen through breath control.

Breath Control is relaxing and places you in the rhythm of the universe. You achieve this by breathing slower, longer and manipulating breath in retention, inhale and exhale.

The first lesson in Pranayama is to take your pulse and divide by ten and this is your universal rhythm. Here you tune into the stars in the galaxies as well as the energy at the core of the earth both which have immense energy that is chemically synthesized into nutrition and reaches through the plants that breathe giving us nutrition to aid in our energy and metamorphosis.

Take your pulse and for demonstration we will say its 60 seconds. Do this by feeling with your index and middle fingers placed on your wrist or neck. Count for 1 minute and then divide by ten. This is your universal rhythm and in this case is 6. To apply this breath in for 6 seconds, hold for 6 seconds and breathe out for 6 seconds. As you practice this during yoga positions or Asanas it will aid in concentration of the exercise benefiting the body for detoxing.

There is an advanced method of this that is called Retention Breathing where you sit or stand increasing the inhalation to 24 seconds and hold for 64 and then exhale for 36. This is called Kumbaka or retention in San Skrit.

Kumbhaka Pranayama: *"He obtains the position of Raja Yoga undoubtedly. Kundalini awakens by Kumbhaka, and by its awakening, Susumna becomes free from impurities."* Gita

"Kumbhaka is the keeping the air confined inside. Rechaka is expelling the confined air. The instructions for Puraka (inhale), Kumbhaka and Rechaka will be found at the proper place and it should be carefully followed. By drawing up from below (Mula Bandha) and contracting the throat (Jalanddhara Bandha) and by pulling back the middle of the front portion of the body (i.e., belly), the Prana goes to the Brahma Nadi (Susumna)". Gita

Monier-Williams defines the compound prāṇāyāma as (m., also pl.) "N. of the three 'breath-exercises' performed during Saṃdhyā (See pūraka, recaka, kumbhaka"

This technical definition refers to a particular system of breath control with three processes as explained by Bhattacharyya: pūraka (to take the breath inside), kumbhaka (to retain it), and recaka (to discharge it). There are also other processes of pranayama in addition to this three-step model." Wikipedia; Pranayama

"By means of various postures and different Kumbhakas, when the great power (Kundali) awakens, then the Prana becomes absorbed in Sunya (Void)." Gita This verse shows the importance of Pranayama for the energy of Kundalini and the absorption into bliss, one with god.

The pranayama breathing exercises are vital to your life. Pranayama (vital force) awakens Shakti (power), frees from disease, detaches you from the world and produces bliss .The respiration, inspiration and the retention will increase in time for each performance. Yoga uses a scale from easy to hard as follows; Adhama – inferior, Madhyama – middle and Uttama – best.

The stages are measured with the performance of Puraka (inspiration), Recaka (expiration) and Kumbhaka (retention). The value is calculated by the length of then PURAKA, KUMBHAKA, and RECAKA.

That is <u>inhaling</u>, <u>retention</u> and <u>exhaling</u>. In that order the assigned values are in seconds;

Adhama   4, 16, and 8 = 28

Madhyama   8, 32, and 16 = 56

Uttama   *16, 64, and 32 = 112*

As you practice the yogis say that the Adhama causes perspiration and tremors. In Madhyama and Uttama, when done a 100 times, produces levitation. These pranayama exercises help cleanse the central nervous system. This then creates a fire that rises from the root chakra awakening

When you breathe it is best to not practice with short breath limiting oxygen intake. When you breath use the Diaphragm, a muscle between the spine and esophagus, by pressing the muscle towards the spine while exhaling and away while inhaling. This is Diaphragm Breathing that athletes and singers practice to extend performance. Likewise, this will enhance the length of your breathing for exercising more efficient.

Physiology of Pranayama by Dr. M. Hajirnis, Thane:

"The process of respiration has three components. Pooraka is inspiration of air, kumbhaka means retention, and rechaka is expiration. It can be said that kumbhaka is pranayama and pranayama is kumbhaka, not pooraka and rechaka, which are natural processes. Kumbhaka is again of three types. Bahir kumbhaka is retention of breath at the end of expiration. Antar kumbhaka means holding the breath after inspiration of air, and kevala kumbhaka or sahaja kumbhaka implies holding the

breath with no particular state of respiration in consideration. *Kevala kumbhaka* is one of the final stages of yoga parallel with the state of *samadhi*. *Bahir kumbhaka* is not used very often. Hence we shall consider *antar kumbhaka* i.e. retention or holding the breath after fully inspiring or taking in air.

What happens in kumbhaka

The physicochemical process of diffusion is dependent mostly on the extent of surface area available for the process to take place, the condition of the membrane in between, and the pressure of gases on either side of the membrane. The process of diffusion, especially of gases as occurs in respiration, is not so much dependent on the time factor. Once the pressure of gases is equalized on either side of the membrane, diffusion comes to a standstill. Hence, withholding the breath for a longer time does not afford any advantage as far as the exchange of gases is concerned. What then could be the advantages derived from *kumbhaka*?

The rate of the heart is slowed in inspiration. With a slower rate, the resting period of the heart- the diastole- is prolonged. Not only does the heart muscle receive more rest, but the cavities of the heart are also better filled with blood. During the next pumping *action of contraction (systole), more blood is pushed into circulation with a better force. Thus general circulation is improved.*

During kumbhaka no new air is entering the lungs, so no more oxygenation is taking place. The oxygen tension in the blood is reduced. Up to a certain level this has an advantage. The brain is most sensitive to this lowered oxygen tension, as its needs for oxygen are the greatest. If the quality of the blood is below par, the brain tries to get more blood in quantity.

In the brain and even elsewhere in the body, all the capillaries are not functioning at all times. Some of them are lying dormant in a collapsed or closed state. In order to receive a greater quantity of blood, these capillaries are opened up. The effect is more marked in the brain. Thus cerebral anoxia leads to cerebral vasodilation, more capillaries open up and circulation improves.

It must be emphasized that this effect is beneficial up to a certain optimum level only. Beyond this level it is distinctly harmful. Hence, it is always stressed that the practice of kumbhaka must be undertaken with the guidance of an experienced teacher. The practice of pranayama has fallen into disrepute in the eyes of the public, mainly because of the malpractice of breath retention. This explanation of cerebral anoxia, causing cerebral vasodilation, applies equally well to the practice of bahir kumbhaka.

Slow Rechaka

The third phase of respiration is expiration. Expiration is a passive act. For stretching a rubber band one needs a conscious effort, while once the active action is released the rubber automatically assumes its original position. The same principle applies to the act of respiration. But the yogic act of rechaka is a slow, guided and controlled process. It should take double the time taken for inspiration.

The first advantage of slow respiration is mechanical. With a sudden release the rubber or the elastic tissue in the lungs will snap back violently, but with a slow release it will maintain its elasticity. The major advantage of slow rechaka, however, is in the brain and psyche. The conscious effort required for slow release needs the help of the cerebral cortex of the brain. The cerebral cortex sends inhibitory impulses to the respiratory centre in the midbrain. These inhibitory impulses from the cortex overflow into the adjoining area of the hypothalamus concerned with emotions, and quieten this area. Hence, the soothing effect of a slow expiration.

It also helps the next stage of ashtanga yoga i.e. pratyahara. Pratyahara means drawing in of the senses and the thought processes. The human mind is like a child. If it is asked not to do a certain thing, it will deliberately try to do it. Hence it is better to give a positive suggestion to a child as well as to the human mind. Instead of asking it to stop thinking, it is given the positive suggestion of observing the respiration. Thus the senses and the thought processes are automatically switched off.

Throughout our life, we are breathing continuously, and involuntarily, day in and day out, during waking and sleeping states. The very first instruction in the teaching of pranayama is to observe this breathing process as it is going on naturally, without trying to modify it. Even this simple act has a physiological implication. Automatic respiration is controlled by the respiratory centre, situated in the midbrain. But once we become aware of the process of respiration, its control shifts to the cerebral cortex. This involvement of the cerebral cortex causes the cortex to develop. Further development of the cerebral cortex leads to a higher stage of the evolutionary cycle."

http://www.yogamag.net/archives/1983/ajan83/physpran.shtml

Diaphragm Breathing

Pranayama means breath control taken in a direction. Diaphragm breathing is the correct way to fill your lungs properly. The ancient translation reads that Prana, which dwells in the heart, draws Apana, which dwells in the Muladhara (root chakra) and Apana draws Prana, a falcon attached by a string is drawn back again when he attempts to fly. This is a colorful expression of diaphragm breathing. The diaphragm is a muscle between the stomach and the esophagus.

The breathing control is to expand the lower lung by pushing the diaphragm out to fill the lungs from the bottom to the top and then pushing the diaphragm towards the spine to empty the lungs. When you fill a pitcher with water the bottom is filled first. The diaphragm is a muscle and this control will help strengthen the belly. This will increase the oxygen throughout all of your body dramatically. The air we breathe is the same energy that inspires all physical matter and releases tension. During the Hath-Yoga postures breath control is done rhythmically.

1. Inhale pushing the diaphragm away from the spine

2. Exhale pushing diaphragm muscle towards the spin

3. Place your hand on your stomach and notice the breath direction

The breath control that reaches higher levels has an astounding effect on the brain with an octave higher resonance in the skull that releases endocrine secretions of glandular sources such as pineal and pituitary. This function excites chemical electrical pathways throughout the two hemispheres of the brain. The brain has regional spikes for processing information. The Pranayama expands at trillions of points promoting bliss on a grand scale with spikes of energy.

As you practice and develop breath control you will increase oxygen, which breaks down matter for energy, 24/7 365 days a year. Each involuntary breath brings in more oxygen for healthy results and this multiplies the benefits of Pranayama dramatically. The volume of oxygen increases the breakdown of matter in your body as it does in nature where biodegradable actions are universal for energy. The more energy you have the healthier you are. A tree produces an apple from the minerals and radiant sunlight and when it ripens it falls to the earth and biodegrades returning ripe and naturally sweetened nutrition to the earth in a cycle of consumption and production. Likewise, in your body as you consume biodegradable nutrients you produce energy as the minerals ripen into protein sugars called amino acids that give you energy.

The Sun's radiation and the oxygen we breathe have grown all of the earth and space we live in is a constant respiration that breaks down matter creating energy. To exist in time and space equilibrium of balanced energy must exist. The universe is expanding as we dwell in our space. Breath control helps us feel the pulse of this vast universe. Because oxygen is the creation of life and the Sun's energy is the radiant light that fuses with the world, life is created. The forces of this light and power of energy from respiration to break down the matter of creation make life possible. Here we breathe for life and introspection of this phenomenon will enlighten us physically and spiritually. When we feel the effects of the natural power at work from the inner self and in the outer universe there is a rhythm that encompasses our thoughts and feelings and increased breath control multiplies this bliss as we connect to a universal connection that makes us one in the energy of the universe. Here there is pure energy and cannot receive judgements but uniqueness of Christ consciousness without judging. Here we are in pure energy and the development of this calm us with peace of the light it amplifies in an Aura visible by photo of light spectrum capabilities.

There are many types of Pranayama practices and know it is an essential pillar of the yoga process.

The Breath of Fire – Bhastrika

Bhastrika, in Sanskrit, means bellow breathing because it is like a bellow that you use to blow on a fire in a pump action to energize the fire with oxygen. After you have learned diaphragm breathing you will increase the intensity to rapid breath in and out of fire as in the fireside pumping the bellows.

When you blow on a fire oxygen with carbons from your body it helps ignite the fire that produces embers into the air that are consumed by oxygen. This is a rapid process of fire starting. With the Breath of Fire, you internally increase the molecular combustion of breakdown and buildup of nutrients for consumption and production of energy.

"Hydroxylation is a chemical process that introduces a hydroxyl group (-OH) into an organic compound. In biochemistry, hydroxylation reactions are often facilitated by enzymes called hydroxylases. Hydroxylation is the first step in the oxidative degradation of organic compounds in air. It is extremely important in detoxification since hydroxylation converts lipophilic compounds into water-soluble (hydrophilic) products that are more readily excreted." Wikipedia Hydroxylation

This explains that water that is 2 parts hydrogen and 1 part oxygen, H_2O, is mixed with organic compounds of minerals and vitamins. When we breath in and out the toxins are removed from the body through circulation and respiration. Rapid *movement of this increases the detoxifying process oxidative degradation into water soluble products that we excrete through breathing.*

When you learn diaphragm manipulation of breath control and fill your lungs with air from the bottom up and not from the top that robs your body of necessary oxygen and can cause hyper ventilation. The movement of in and out from the spine done slowly can be increased to a rapid pace creating a fanning of the fire as well as strengthening the stomach muscle or the diaphragm muscle.

Sitting in a comfortable position start the slow in and out from the spine breath control. Increase till you sound like a train and execute this as long as you can. This will increase the release of endocrine secretions giving a blissful feeling. If you are dizzy the other factor is that you are not diaphragm breathing and the short breath is not oxygen rich but oxygen poor so practice deep breathing till your detoxification process is better. The dizziness can also be because toxins that produce phlegm are present in your blood and purification will allow the increased respiration to flow without inhibition.

The effect of this over extended period of time will accelerate the central nervous system chemical electrical rapid signaling of additional oxygen bringing blissful feeling leaving you relaxed. The body has a reward system for eating and sleeping and that is serotonin that is sent from the pineal gland as a byproduct of melatonin or

DMT that is also known as the dream giver. The serotonin is sent as a neurotransmitter to receptors in the guts. Here, after we consume food it produces euphoria for feeding that supports the metabolic functions of your body. These receptors are where they discovered the natural process and synthesized pills like valium and other relaxing medication. With breathing exercises, we stimulate endocrine excretions that relax us like a good meal does.

Yogi Bahjan in Kundalini Yoga says "The focal point of Breath of Fire is on the navel point. The breath is fairly rapid (2 to 3 times a second with practice). It is continuous and powerful with no pause between inhalation and exhalation. Breathe through the nose, unless otherwise directed. Here is how it works: As you inhale the exhale the air is pushed out by pulling the navel point and abdomen towards the spine. As you inhale, release the inward pull of the navel to allow the breath to automatically return to the lungs. It may be helpful at first to put the hand on the abdomen to feel the inward pull on the exhalation, and the subsequent relaxation of the abdomen on the inhalation. Listen to the sound of the breath, which will create the sound of a steam engine.

When inhalation and exhalation are performed very quickly, like a pair of bellows of a blacksmith, it dries up all the disorders from the excess of phlegm, and is known as Kapala Bhati." This is Hindi for couple flows.

Breath of Fire Benefits

1. Cleanses then lungs, cells and blood of toxic waste

2. Increases oxygen intake

3. Strengthens the central nervous system

4. Warms you up

5. Desired effect is accelerated

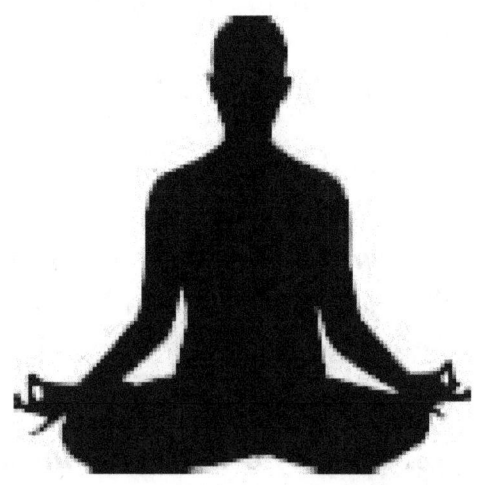

Alternate Sinus Breathing

This is the most popular of all breathing techniques and is a very relaxing and sinus effective breath control. This is the most widely used breath control and is very relaxing

"If the air be inhaled through the left nostril, it should be expelled again through the other, and filling it through the right nostril, confining it there, it should be expelled through the left nostril. By practicing in this way, through the right and the left nostrils alternately, the whole of the collection of the nadis of the yamis (practisers) becomes clean, i.e., free from impurities, after 3 months and over". The Gita

The Nadis is the central nervous system that travels along the spinal column up and down and are filled with energy in sectors called Chakras.

Alternate breathing is breath through alternate nostrils and is done in the easy pose (Sukhasana) or lotus pose (Pdhasana). It is also referred to as Nadi Shuddhi or cleansing of the central nervous system. The alternate nostrils are closed by the right hand using the ring finger, little finger and the thumb. The little finger and ring finger press the left nostril closed and the thumb closes the right nostril. The index finger and the middle finger are placed between the eyebrows where Anja chakra or third eye is. You breathe only through the nose and silently breathe as follows.

The right nostril is closed with the thumb. Air is exhaled through the left nostril, and inhaled back through the same nostril.

The left nostril is closed with the ring finger. Air is exhaled through the right nostril, and inhaled back through the same nostril. This is done with regular breathing and the exhale can be longer than the inhale a ratio of 1:2.

You can hold between breaths or hold for a deeper effect as follows:

Clear your nose. Put your right hand up to your nose. Place your index and middle finger on your forehead, with the thumb and ring finger on either side of your nose.

1. Now use your thumb to close your right nostril. Take a slow, deep breath in through your left nostril, counting 6 to 8 seconds. Slow down your in-breath so that it takes 6 to 8 seconds to fill your lungs.

2. Plug your left nostril (both sides blocked now) and hold your breath to a count of 6 to 8.

3. Now lift your thumb off your right nostril (keep left nostril closed) and breathe out, through your right nostril only, for a count of 6-8.

4. Do not pause at the end of the breath. Start breathing in through the right nostril to a count of eight.

5. Plug both sides and hold breath for a count 6 to 8.

6. Now breathe out through your left nostril for a count of eight.

7. Continue to breathe in and out through alternate nostrils:

IN the left HOLD

OUT the right HOLD

IN the right HOLD

OUT the left HOLD

IN the left HOLD

When you are breathing and holding there is a rhythm that is personal to you and this called Rhythmic Breathing. Take your pulse for one minute and divide it by six. The pulse can be found in the neck and wrist. When breathing in or out count the pulse rate calculation for each breath. If it is 60 then six counts to each inspiration and expiration. With time the rhythm will increase as your breathing improves through the vital force practice. As you perform the paced breathing will aid you in concentration and focusing on the breath of life or Pranayama. As the Kumbhaka, or retention breathing, it is increased in time the rhythm will be extended to 10, 11 and more.

For thousands of years we have danced and chanted with rhythm. Under the majestic sky filled with constellations to the fire light that warmed and sparkling legends. The

Native Americans Pow Wows are colorful display and the totem poles are considered by some as energy centers in hierarchy of animal glyphs. The dancing and rhythm of this culture is mesmerizing as they interpret the heavens with ancestors from the starry world where they watch from and embody the dancers in shamanistic way to heal the community. Our bodies have an internal clock and this constitutes a set rhythm for sleeping and waking. Endocrine glands aid us with dream secretions at sunset. Others control eating habits. Our pulse rate is what determines the rhythm during Asanas. It is important that you do the breathing with rhythm. This is your relationship to the rhythm of the world. It helps you focus and relax as well as initiates oxygen rejuvenation for your respiratory system and a basic key to breathing performance. Your body is in rhythm with the universe and the breathing will match this rhythm along with your personal signature.

The respiratory system is dynamically improved with the breathing techniques. The sinus cavity and the olfactory bulb at the base of the brain receive a healthy dose of oxygen. The olfactory bulb is filled with sensory transmitters and communicates with the hippocampus as well as other parts of the brain. The release of GABA gamma-Aminobutyric acid is an stimulated action. "The main observation was that in the hippocampus and neocortex of the mammalian brain, GABA has primarily excitatory effects, and is in fact the major excitatory neurotransmitter in many regions of the brain."- Wikipedia-GABA. GABA relaxes the sinus area and is one of the main nuropeptides that enhance relaxation in the brain. When the pranayama process is established with practice this excited the release of GABA. With the healthy breath control and the interaction with space drawing in oxygen at an increased controlled level will initiate a response from the bodily functions. This will be evident as the mucus of the sinus cavity clears. You will be able to feel this tingling fresh sensation in your sinus as the flow of oxygen and blood excite the transmission of neurotransmitters to enhance the nasal area. The freshness of air coming from space interacting with the neurotransmitters will open a new world of understanding your inner self. The direct transmission between the olfactory bulb (smelling) and hippocampus (brain section for memory) is what gives you memory of the fresh smell of flowers. The excitement of this feeling and the increased levels of mood enhancing secretions on the central nervous system will revive a freshness right where the life force enters your body. The clearing of the nasal cavity and reduction of swelling to restrict air flow will be the benefit of the breath control process. This is very effective to promote health of the cognitive skills as the oxygen that enters the nose is directly connected to the brain region that governs memory. It is the physical detrition of the hippocampus that Alzheimer's disease and other cognitive skills are caused.

During my research I came upon a breathing exercise that was a very vigorous and effective exercise that is dynamic for your respiratory strength and vitality. I call this exercise Hatha Pranayama or Sun Moon Breath Control.

This breath control is ancient and a wonderful breath control that will invigorate and stimulate the energy in your body.

1. Standing spread your feet and extend your arms at an angle above your head, like a jumping jack and stretch your arms outwards. Rise up on your toes while stretching and breathe in, bring arms down and exhale. Repeat 3 times.

Stand with your feet together and extend your hands out in front of you and palms together. Move them with inhaling and moving them rhythmically from the middle and move the arms extending from the shoulders and back to the middle exhaling. Repeat 5 times with rhythm. This is known as Bhastrika method of breathing through the nose with equal time for inhalation and exhalation. The purpose is to execute the breath longer and deeper with equal time intervals that soothe and relax you. This is Bhastrika Pranayama. With practice you will breathe inward and outward at longer intervals. Feel the stillness and quiet rhythm that grows in you. Yogis call this the ocean breath.

2. Cleansing Breath

Note the cleansing breath is when you have held your breath then release by creasing your tongue and blowing out in short burst using diaphragm muscle. It will take three or four bursts. This will allow the toxins from oxygen breakdown to be expelled.

Standing inhale, diaphragm to fill from the bottom, and exhale in spurts without your cheeks puffing out. Empty your lungs and push the abdomen towards the spine pushing the air out. This will help clear your lungs over time and help clean the throat and esophagus.

3. Standing in mountain pose extend your arms to the side, from the shoulders, inhale and hold. Then rotate in small circles comfortably. (15-60 seconds)

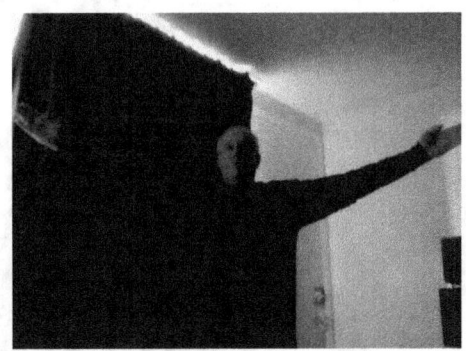

4. Standing inhale and extend arms out from body and clench fists. Grip tensely, move at a rapid pace back to your chest and out again. Hold for however you can be comforted, do not push. First time try 20 seconds. Increase as you practice to 1 minute.

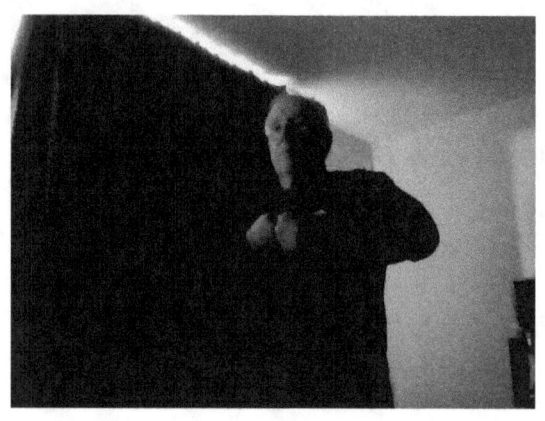 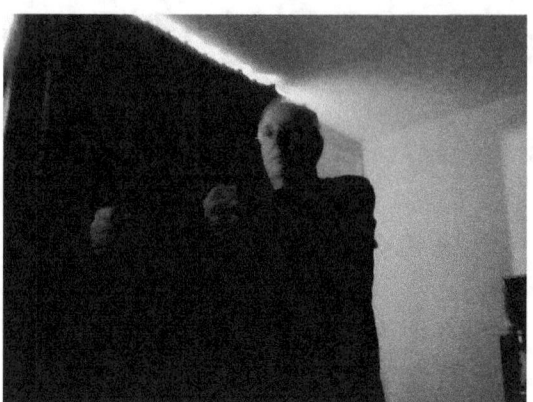

5. Cleansing Breath

6. Standing inhale and extend arms straight out from shoulder, clench fists and rapidly move to your chest and back for comfortable amount of time. (15 to 60 seconds)

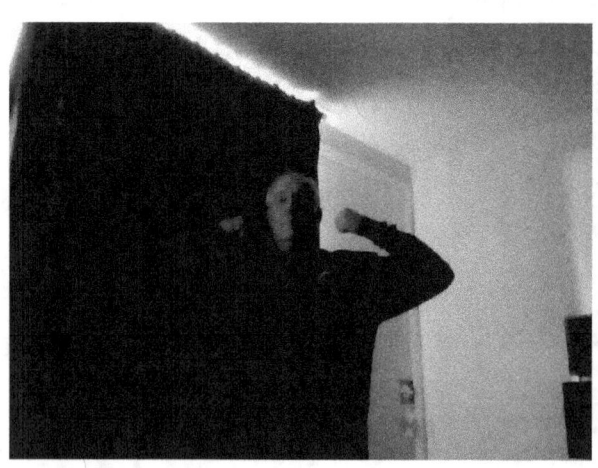 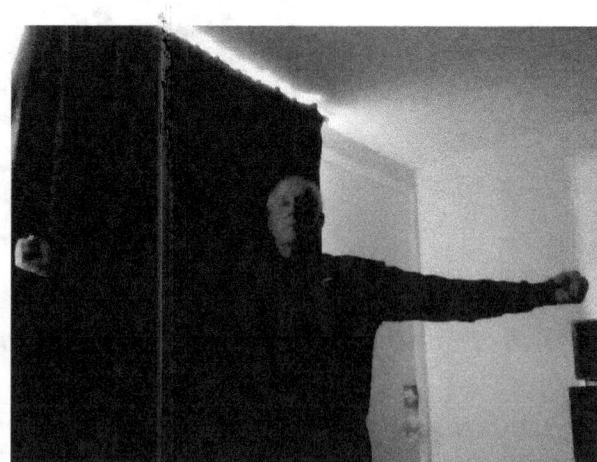

7. Cleansing Breath

8. Standing inhale and grip your chest by putting your thumbs in your arm pits and fingers wrapped around your chest and squeeze and hold comfortably.

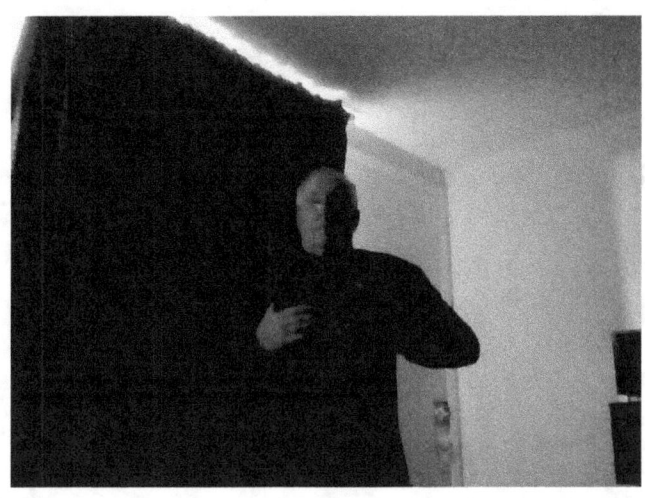

9. Cleansing Breath

10. Inhale and hold while tapping on your chest with finger to help stimulate blood and healing. Finish using palms for tapping.

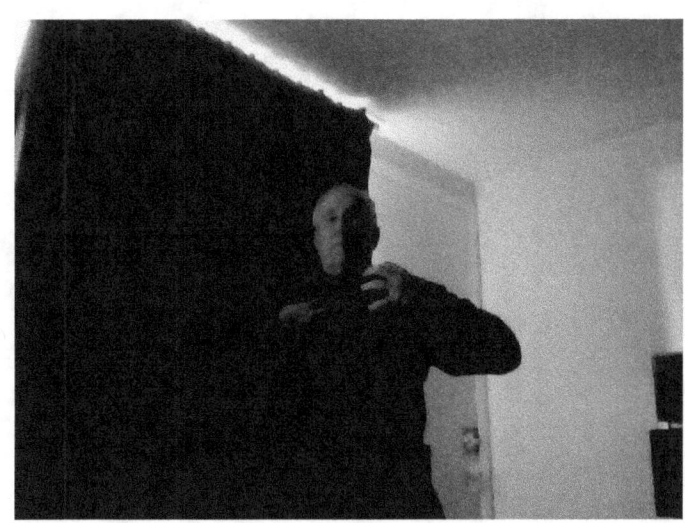

11. Cleansing Breath

Relax and feel the oxygen at work throughout the body, this is an ancient technique of Hatha-Yoga in Pranayama or breath control.

I practice this daily along with retention breathing and it increases my respiration dynamically like a runner.

Chapter 7. Energy

What this whole book and my former books is about is energy. The food we eat, the sun we get, the exercising we do and the breath control we practice gives us energy.

In the hunter and gatherer stage we were active and eating fresh game and nuts, berries and fish. Nature has a balance that is energy expanding in the universe and the micro inner world of our cells. In time and space this equilibrium is a balance of energy that when is bright and flowing is disease free.

The yoga process is unification of body and mind. From the beginning we developed the feeding parts (gastrointestinal) and then connected to the brain making a genetic chain of energy to the cognitive skills to survive by hunting and gathering for food. The less we learn to survive on the pillars of immunity and the more convenient we allow production of unhealthy metabolic behavior to exist our body will dissipate energy. Conversely, nutrition of fresh minerals and vitamins combined with solar radiant energy and aerobic heat that causes chemical synthesis transferring energy we will be vibrant with energy.

The ancient science of the minerals and energy developed a Chakra chart that designated different energy centers from the base of the spine to the crest of the head. This information from early medical researchers manipulated breath and chemical-

electrical spinal connection along the spine to the brain establishing a spinal-cerebral super connectivity. This connectivity increases the flow of Central Nervous System electrical energy between synapse and dendrite that is the male and female plugs between molecules that produce proteins that are the basis of energy production.

The more energy you have the better you feel. So the energy and breath control exercises dynamically improve energy by increasing oxygen, a biodegradable function that breaks down matter for production of energy from consumption of nutrients and Body Locks, discussed further, that redistribute neurotransmitters to the cognitive process. This is what Einstein was referring to when he said we have a servant and a master. The master is our inner self energy of light that can open and enlighten the creative powers of the brain. The creativity is what machines will never do no how many robots they invent. Also, there is no drug that can relax and give you positive vibes in perfect balance of cognitive creativity.

This ancient science developed a system they called Kundalini and based is neurotransmitter findings on writings over 4000 years ago. The early writings talked of the spinal connections and Kundalini practitioners applied pressure on the spine with the diaphragm muscle that is positioned between the stomach and the spine, a Body Lock. When this is done the negative and positive electrical transmissions governing our behavior and functions reverse, partially, the electrical transmission back to the brain electrifying multiple regions of the brain bring an incredible cranial tingling that releases serotonin and other endocrine or inner secretions of metabolic

transmitters.

Serotonin is a neurotransmitter released as a byproduct from the pineal gland of DMT or the dream secretion. This neurotransmitter travels from the pineal to the gastrointestinal regions signaling satisfaction for consuming food. That "Ah" feeling after you eat a good meal. Therefore, the reversal of this flow returns the serotonin giving a blissful feeling and producing alpha waves of balance and euphoria.

The connectivity from the gastrointestinal region to the brain is a spinal-cerebral flow and in the middle of the back is a relay station that sends energy to the horse tail that has 72000 nerves spreading out to the base of the spine and to the peripheral areas of the lower body.

Body Locks (Bhandi Locks)

The Bhandi locks stimulate and energize the spine and brain. During this process the Pituitary gland, pineal gland and other glands secrete balancing bodily functions. It is homeostasis functioning for sexual behavior, food intake and many others.

The physiological process opens the path to an intuitive application of the power of sexual behavior and affects a natural balance in both sexes. The ability of nature to balance the forces in us can take addicted behavior and reduce dependency on a multitude of out of balance functions is amazing and can be a part of intervention and rehabilitation efforts with much better results. In our society we take adverse behavior and add to the dilemma by taking nature further away through drugs. This is the very opposite that should be done. Ascend the light within us and without us and the world we will be a brighter place to live. The application of pills put us at risk in our immune system giving rise to physical and psychological disorder.

The energy we perfect through nutritional metabolic safe consumption aids in our physical and mental stability. The energy that is out of balance uses pressure in the body causing brain dysfunctions and need the nutrition and aerobic oxygen to balance out the energy that suffers from acid levels that need alkaline that quells the acrid levels destroying cells and then allows diseases to form and grow. With the energy purification that has writings that go back over 4000 years neutralizes the acids and forming diseases. As detoxing effects are felt the energy is freeing itself of toxins that bog it down and the electrical transmissions are faster and healthier increasing bodily function and cognitive processing. In short you will be sharp as a whip increasing thought process.

To manipulate the cerebral-spinal connections the body locks are performed in the following. For a complete Kundalini Yoga refer to Yoga light featured on my sight www.yogasunmoon.com

Body locks - Bandhas

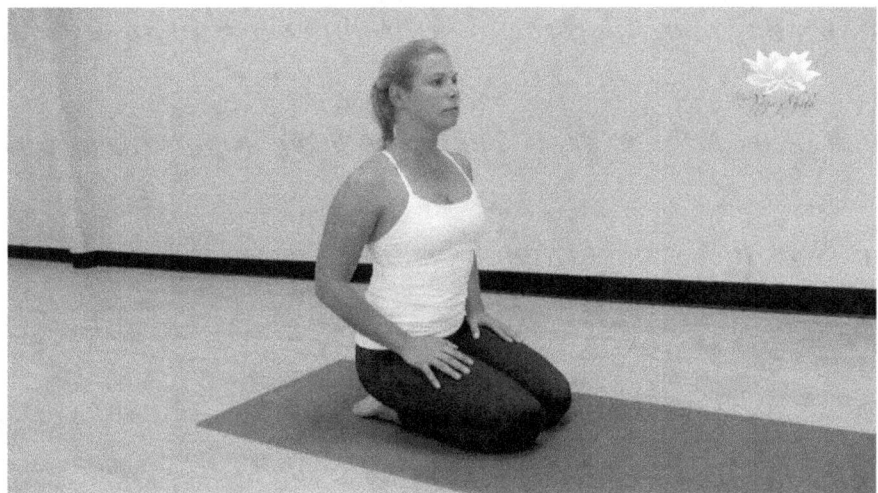

Thunderbolt (Vajrāsana)

The Sanskrit word, Siddha means adept or accomplished. This, in yoga terms, means to be accomplished at perfectly still in the mind.

This posture is referred to as both the stone and thunderbolt. The names both have meaning to Kundalini in the sense that you sit firmly, stone and awaken an electrical surge, thunderbolt that opens bio-dynamic pathways (Nadis and Susumna) through the energy centers or chakras.

In Kundalini Yoga Yogi Bhajan explains "Body locks are certain combinations of muscle contractions. Each lock functions to change blood circulation, nerve activity and the flow of cerebral spinal fluid. They also direct the flow of pranayama, life force to the main energy channels that relate to raising the Kundalini energy. There are three important locks in Kundalini Yoga: Neck lock, Diaphragm lock, and Root lock". Kundalini Yoga p.15

You actually isolate the flow of energy and reverse the electrical channeling that stimulates the cranial and bodily functions. This results in sensational bio-dynamic experience. Through time the energy paths will be efficient and the sensation can be experienced when you cleanse the nadis (spinal nerves) of toxins sensitizing the cerebra-spinal connections.

Neck Lock

Jalahandra Bandh:

Sit in stone position with back straight and exhale completely and contract the neck and throat and hold and lower chin towards the sternum. Hold for as long as it is comfortable and increase to 20 seconds and above with practice. Exhale.

Some yogis prefer keeping head straight to align spine, either way is optional. The Gita says, "It stops the opening (hole) of the group of Nadis, through which the juice from the sky (from the Soma or Chandra in the brain) falls down. It is, therefore, called the Jalandhara Bandha -- the destroyer of a host of diseases of the throat".

Diaphragm Lock

Uddiyana Bandh:

Sit with straight spine empty lungs with exhale. Pull and contract diaphragm back towards spine and upward collapsing the abdomen in and upward. Do this smooth and slow so the muscle does the work. Never force any yoga asana or kriyas. Always stay in comfort zone. The Gita explains "The portions above and below the navel, should be drawn backwards towards the spine. By practicing this for six months one can undoubtedly conquer death."

Root Lock

Mul bandh:

Inhale and contract the anal muscle and put heel, if comfortable, under the rectum. Then draw the diaphragm towards the spine. Hold. Exhale

Yogis report from the Gita, "The Kundalini, which has been sleeping all this time, becomes well heated by this means and awakens well. It becomes straight like a serpent, struck dead with a stick."

The Great Lock

Maha Bandh

Inhale with straight spine. Apply all body locks at once. Start with root and go up to throat and hold comfortably. Gita expresses "Fill in the air, keeping the chin firm against the chest, and, having pressed the air, and the mind should be fixed on the middle of the eyebrows or in the susumna (the spine). This Maha Bandha is the most skillful means for cutting away the snares of death."

You will gradually couple with purification and exercise feel the energy centers awaken. This will tap into the body natural stress relief and stimulation of cranial creativity the abdomen, heart, rectum and esophagus to throat will be stimulated with oxygen and circulatory improvements along with the energy centers awakened.

Practice with caution because if you are filled with toxins there will be dizziness until you have detoxed. However, this exercise is the best for stimulating connections in the nasal area promoting open sinus that Sudafed and Claritin have analyzed and synthesized into sinus and allergy pills.

As I have said the energy manipulation of the energy centers are the Chakras. They are famous for the third eye and here in meditation the energy is concentrated on the vast universe of the inner self.

People tend to think that as we walk along the path of life that we are separated and superior to nature. In ancient timed the environment was a survival against the elements and predators like tigers and lions. The philosophers that dealt with this problem spoke of two things. One the dominance of the wild and the honoring of that which they saw in nature. We have strayed away and have chased many animals into extinction and nature into concrete and steel. But, we are an inseparable part of nature.

There is a law that governs us each day and night and that is physics. We are organisms that have evolved from solar radiation, bacterial synthesis and oxygen regeneration and the whole planet is in this life cycle. We are part of nature and that is why organic nutrition works so well for health and metabolic functions.

"The metabolism of an organism determines which substances it finds nutritious and which it will find poisonous. For example, some prokaryotes (bacteria) use hydrogen sulfide as a nutrient, yet this gas is poisonous to animals. The speed of metabolism, the metabolic rate, influences how much food an organism will require, and also affects how it is able to obtain that food.

A striking feature of metabolism is the similarity of the basic metabolic pathways and components between even vastly different species. For example, the set of that are best known as the intermediates in the citric acid cycle are present in all known organisms, being found in species as diverse as the unicellular bacteria Escherichia coli and huge multicellular organisms like elephants. These striking similarities in metabolic pathways are likely due to their early appearance in evolutionary history, and being retained because of their efficacy." Ebenhöh O, Heinrich R (2001). *"Evolutionary optimization of metabolic pathways. Theoretical reconstruction of the stoichiometry of ATP and NADH producing systems". Bull Math Biol 63 (I): 21–55. doi:10.1006/bulm.2000.0197. PMID 11146883.*

When we cook a sauce we put spices in to enhance flavor.to do this we simmer in a low heat for spices to blend or bind chemically. When we eat this is the same process. Our digestive system releases 50% of what we eat half for nature and half for us. This is subdivided more into energy for our daily needs as calories to think and exist running our functions. This 50% of the remaining 50% allotted for daily needs. The other half is in storage for work and hunting and gathering food for survival. This is there and if not used becomes sedentary and turns to fat. So 25% of the mineral value of nutrition is not used to build healthy tissue and energy to create a strong immune system.

When we look deeply inside to the inner self we are scientists with a vested interest in our health only. Here the Third Eye is a looking glass that connects to the multiple regions of the brain and stimulate thinking that stimulates the hemispheric health of the brain. When we sleep we go thru REM, Rapid Eye Movement, and this is a tune up of free thinking without any outside direction and some very crazy zany geams occur. Some of these dreams have produced mathematical wonders and creative media by artist. Here creativity abounds. Likewise, when we meditate the Hippocampus that controls our memory to navigate in our environment. Attached to that are two brain areas the olfactory and amygdala. The olfactory is the sinus where oxygen, the vital force, enters and we use to scent things and identify what we scent with the memory like a rose or a skunk. The amygdala is the fight and flight for danger and survival.

When you meditate the hippo campus grows throughout your life giving good memory and steady thinking. When you are scared and have anxiety the amygdala increases in size and conversely when you meditate this brain function shrinks. So meditation is deep and healthy practice and use of your energy.

To meditate closing your eyes and transfix your mind on the energy within you and here there is a judge not freedom that relaxes you as natural where you are perfect when you leave the world of temptations by concentrating upon the energy of your body. This is a light that shines inside and outside in what is called an aura. This is the Chakra Aura and is the eighth chakra. Here are the most known and practiced chakras listed here for your understanding.

Ancient Chakras of Cosmic Energy

Kundalini Yoga is ancient wisdom for the piercing of energy centers or Chakras. We all have auras and this light from electromagnetic light waves is most bright when the Chakras are stimulated. This has been said by a clairvoyant that can perceive light beyond the normal perception. Yoga Light explains, instructs and shows how to pierce the Chakras of ancient wisdom to awaken the resting energy into a rising energy propelled like a rocket in a cerebral-spinal flash. This is what Einstein has proved and what the Kundalini Yoga has disciplined.

There are 8 Chakras including the Aura Chakra. Through the yoga process you can feel the energy that ascends through the body enlightening and awakening energy. The Crown Chakra is at the top of the head and trillions of connections passing neurotransmitter information dazzle your brain producing strong Alpha waves of electromagnetic wave lengths. Here is where the detachment and transcendental phenomenon absorbs into the true self. Here, "Like a child", we absorb into the Supreme Self detached from temporal distraction or temptation of the world.

The Third Eye or Ajna Chakra is between the eyebrows and you can feel the energy as you use the Kundalini Body Locks. The energy ascends to the Crown after the Third Eye.

The Seven Energy Centers/Chakras

8. Aura   *Inner/Outer Light*

7. Sahasrara: *Crown Chakra*

6. Ajna: *Brow Chakra*

5. Vishuddha: *Throat Chakra*

4. Anahata: *Heart Chakra*

3. Manipura: *Solar Plexus Chakra*

2. Swadhisthana: *Sacral Chakra*

1. Muladhara: *Root Chakra*

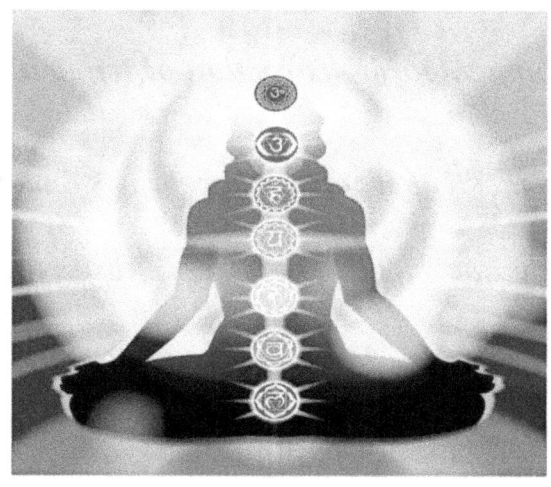

From the base of spine where 7200 nerves stretch out the energy rises through the cerebra-spinal system (Nadis) connecting key elements of electrical pathways to brain functions aided by oxygen circulated by the heart to the molecular level of the brain where energy excites endocrine glands to secrete anxiety reducing and blissful enhancement

neurotransmitter ionized (combustion and conductivity) information throughout the brain. This is a physiological reality that when the brain is stimulated the meditative practice is enhanced and other areas of the brain are affected and trillions of connections are energized awakening the psycho-spiritual transcendental illumination.

8. Aura Chakra *is the light from within emitting out of your body. The more energy from purification the brighter the Aura.*

7. Sahasrara Chakra *(Crown energy center) is located at the top of the head and encompasses both hemispheres of the brain like a crown of electricity arcing plasma reaching out in a spectacular connection combining the endocrine gland transmissions on a natural level and non-regional spikes of electrical-chemical transmissions at trillions of locations.*

6. Ajna Chakra *(Third Eye energy center) is located between the eyebrows and cultivates visions with the energy stimulating the pineal* and assimilating thyroid and pituitary electrical transmissions.*

5. Vishuddha Chakra *(Throat Chakra energy center) is located in the throat and lower back of head and its secretions are tied with the Moon Chakra or Bindu Chakra and stimulates the pituitary and thyroid endocrine glands.*

4. *Anahata Chakra* *(Heart Chakra energy center) is the heart chakra that is the respiratory and circulation of pranayama (Vital force of Breath).*

3. *Manipura Chakra* *(Solar Plexus energy center) is located at the solar plexus near 4th vertebrae of back where the filum terminale** of the central nervous system is felt that energizes the Kundalini Shakti upward and energy is highly cognitive during arousal and manifests at the solar plexus region being propelled by the cerebral-spinal excitement of the cauda equina. This area is filled with vitality and is prominent with pranayama activity and has grey matter in spinal fluids.*

2. *Swadhisthana Chakra* *(Sacral Chakra energy center) position is stimulated by the cauda equina*** where 72000 nerves spread out like a horse tail that are receiving the root chakra awakening and propelling the energy up the spine to this location.*

1. *Muladhara Chakra* *(Root Chakra energy center) is at the rectal area where the nerve system is highly sensitive with 72000 nerves surrounding and is awakened on the journey through the energy centers.*

* Pineal Gland located between hemispheres of brain secreting melatonin and serotonin

** Filum Terminale thread like nerve connecting lower back of 72000 A terminal conjoining brain and gastrointestinal regions.

*** Cauda Equina base of spine where 72000 nerves spread out like a horse tail

The electrical energy that is resurrected and then multiplied through muscular manipulations infuse the brain with additional blood past the blood barrier into the brain that soaks up the nutrition and delivers biodynamic activity that is expressed as ten million lightning's as a description of the tingling effect of the energy surge in the brain.

The scientific discoveries have underlined the electrical-chemical process by identifying spikes of encoded energy that communicate to the intracellular cranial network in fields of data recognition that then send the information to the upper brain for interpretation. The yoga excites trillions of connections not specific fields of thinking ability but throughout the base then the higher regions in both hemispheres creating a phenomenal electrical surge of billions and trillions of spikes. This then enhances functions of glandular transmissions to stabilize, visualize and balance biological phenomenon. It "shines like a chain of lightning flashes". Gita.

The energy that is awakened travels the spinal columns central nervous system and with muscle contractions reverses the electrical flow down the spine in an upward direction. The first contraction of Bindu Locks is the Root Bandh and it awakens the CNS and begins the ascension to the higher Chakras. The next sensations you will feel the flow from the spinal base and then powerful energy in the middle back area of the Solar Plexus energy center. Then the Third Eye chakra where the lower regions of the brain where the pineal, thyroid and pituitary are excited to release secretions that relax and create homeostasis activity for functions of the body. This is evident by the thread like tingling that stimulates the bottom regions of the brain that contain trillions of electrical chemicals connections and neurotransmitter systems for cognitive functions. When this energy ascends with practice the electrical energy rises to the crown area as purification of your transmitting apparatus is achieved through diet and exercise. The crown energy center stimulates trillions of connections completing the energy ascension stimulating the balanced chemical electrical cognitive functions. As the purification and pranayama increase the purity of your system the spinal area (Nadis) will become excited in the solar plexus and nasal cavity through the end of the nose. This is a result of the central nervous system connecting from the spine to the nose opening the nostrils and clearing your head.

The spine is reacting to the purification and the accentuation of the connections and the increase in cardio vascular delivery of oxygen create clear pathways for electro-chemical communication. Stimulating these areas through body locks (Bandhi) with pure pathways excite the glandular secretions and spawn's intellectual enlightenment. Attaining this enlightenment will reduce anxiety and rewards will be intuitive and blissful. The psycho-spiritual connection will be a consciousness of abstract and concrete balance and the inner self recognition on a transcendental plane. This connection is enhanced with the body locks and breathing exercises also connect help distribute energy throughout the body which is prime function of our body and is our metabolic job to separate poison from nutrition.

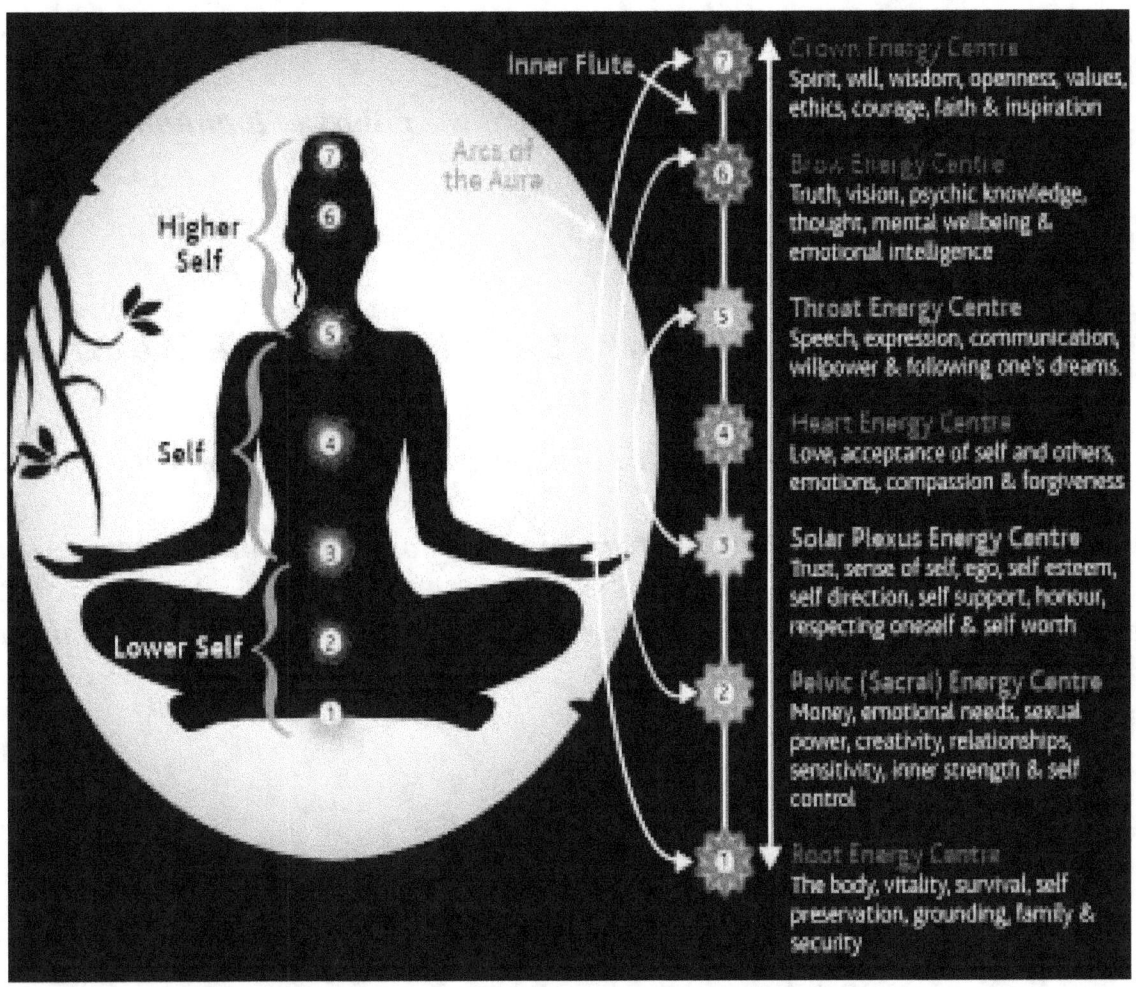

Carl Jung's Chakras with his spiritual sayings that were in the early 20ᵗʰ century

For a complete understanding of yoga process of Kundalini, Hatha and Power Yoga

there are two books for your review at amazon. It can easily be looked at by going to

my site @ www.yogasunmoon.com

The first book is Yoga Light and also Breath of Life is available. Yoga Light is a

comprehensive look at yoga and Kundalini section plus everything you need to begin or review a yoga exercise program. It has been bought by physical therapists for it knowledge and has helped heal people with the three pillars of immunity.

ENERGY IS LIKE A 4 CYLINDER CAR THAT NEEDS FUEL THAT COMBUSTS:

Solar radiation, mineral fuel, oxygen for breaking own matter for energy and aerobic activity to distribute minerals for energy production for regenerating tissue. Thus one cylinder causes energy loss and the engine struggles overworking the other three. It is a question of physics of what is within and without you.

When you eat well but lack aerobic activity the one cylinder is not firing because when you consume food half of it is expelled from the body for soil regeneration as manure of original natural diets and 25% is dispensed for daily requirements and 25% is in reserve for aerobic chemical transfer. When the reserve is not used it is sedentary and if not heated up for energy to transfer into production from consumption of nutrition and sunlight.

The universe was started from energy that was a metamorphic event and produced nutrition the fuel for energy and life itself. When you eat right, think right and feel right it is energy that has enlightened you and it is energy that ascends throughout the

universe.

Summation:

It is survival of the fittest. If you have energy to fight disease you can defeat disease. This is based on the strength of your immunity that depends upon the amount of nutrition, oxygen and sunlight you have plus an aerobic exercise that combines the minerals, radiation and exercise to distribute a fight against poisons. This is what our metabolism is about. It is to separate that which is good and that which is bad before it gets to your body and depletes energy.

Your bloodstream is where the fight goes on. There the Macrophages duel with Nagalese. The nutrition is the fuel for the energy with solar power that consumes and neutralizes the disease that is trying to attack your immunity and neutralize it. The forces are like to prize fighters, one with dead cells rotting and mutating from toxins and the other vibrant solar and mineral energy of living cells.

This is why cancer is an isolated disease when it forms due to a breakdown of cell growth and then it attempts to survive in a mutated state that is toxic to the body.

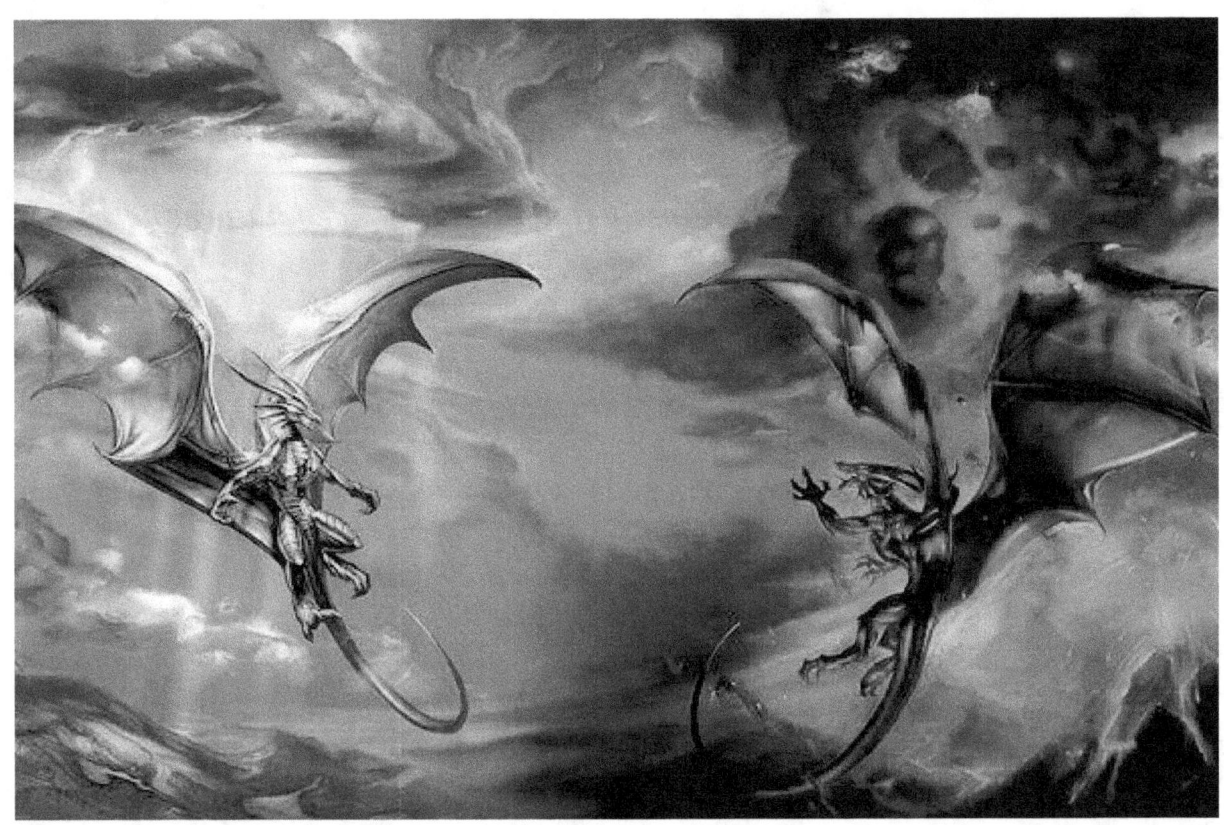

The minerals and vitamins are nature in motion with a harmony and symphony of health that pharmaceuticals can only replicate at higher levels reducing you to dependency without the metabolic power of a stealth fighter to eliminate disease and regenerate the damaged tissue. The metabolic power in our bodies is for our survival and imitation non-organic substitutes do not chemically transfer in an absorption chemical electrical pathways efficient as natural elements. They ride it and cause electrical transfer but at the cost of inhibiting the natural energy consumption of nutrients and production of energy.

All pills are herbal or from nature. You are a part of nature and only nature works on you. Therefore, all pills are synthesized from herbs and plants compounds and reduced to a little pill that takes over your bodily functions that need natural herbs and plants that are fibrous for your body.

The pharmacy is trying to control of your body and yes they can relieve you but it will inhibit your body's natural way of fighting disease and herbs are natural that will heal you without inhibiting your natural functions because they will not addict you by replacing our immune response but enhance your natural body. Fruits and greens have minerals that are the fuel for energy that will give you power for healthy.

Pills drain your energy, and you know this. Plants do not reduce energy and you know this. So increase the plants and reduce the pills till you reduce addiction and then you will not need them and you will not desire them and then the fruits and vegetables will taste great and you will crave natural, fibrous food and this is an energy crave. Do not let the pseudo doctors lie to you anymore. Live to the fullest, richest life. AMEN

"Whole foods — such as fruits, vegetables, grains and dairy

products — have three main benefits you can't get in a pill:

•   Whole foods are complex. They contain a variety of the

nutrients your body needs — not just one. An orange, for

example, provides vitamin C as well as beta carotene,

calcium and other nutrients. Vitamin C supplements

lack these other nutrients. Similarly, a glass of milk

provides you with protein, vitamin D, riboflavin, calcium,

phosphorus and magnesium. If you take only calcium

supplements and skip calcium-rich foods, such as dairy

products, you may miss all the other nutrients you need

for healthy bones.

• *Whole foods provide dietary fiber. Fiber is important for*

digestion, and it helps prevent certain diseases. Soluble

fiber (found in beans, some grains, and some fruits and

vegetables) and insoluble fiber (found in whole grains

and some fruits and vegetables) may help prevent heart

disease, diabetes and constipation.

6 YOUR GUIDE TO VITAMIN & MINERAL SUPPLEMENTS

• *Whole foods contain other substances that may*

be important for good health. Fruits and vegetables,

for example, contain naturally occurring chemicals

(phytochemicals) that may help protect you against major

concerns such as cancer, heart disease, osteoporosis

and diabetes. Although it's not yet known precisely what

role phytochemicals play in nutrition, research shows

many health benefits from eating more fruits, vegetables

and grains. If you depend on supplements rather than

eating a variety of whole foods, you miss the potential

benefits of phytochemicals.

•   *Whole foods contain vitamins in their many forms.*

As mentioned earlier, vitamin A as retinol occurs only in

animal products; plants contain hundreds of carotenoids

that the body can convert into vitamin A.

Concentrate on getting your nutrients from a variety of

foods, not supplements. Whole foods provide an ideal mix

of nutrients, fiber and other food substances." Your Guide to Mineral and Vitamin Supplements,
Mayo Clinic

This underlines the energy is based on fuel from organics that generate energy the

best. They are fibrous and when we break down this matter energy is produced and the metabolic or survival of your body in the world needs this to beam with energy.

The vitamin B12 or protein uses bacteria and archaea that are salt-tolerant archaea (the Haloarchaea) that use sunlight as an energy source, and other species of archaea fix carbon

Vitamin B12 is fermented in the body with a fermentation process "Vitamin B12, vitamin B12 or vitamin B-12, also called cobalamin, is a water-soluble vitamin with a key role in the normal functioning of the brain and nervous system, and for the formation of blood. It is one of the eight B vitamins. It is normally involved in the metabolism of every cell of the human body, especially affecting DNA synthesis and regulation, but also fatty acid metabolism and amino acid metabolism. Neither fungi, plants, nor animals (including humans) are capable of producing vitamin B12. Only bacteria and archaea have the enzymes required for its synthesis, although many foods are a natural source of B12 because of bacterial symbiosis. The vitamin is the largest and most structurally complicated vitamin and can be produced industrially only through bacterial fermentation-synthesis." Yamada, Kazuhiro (2013). "Chapter 9. Cobalt: Its Role in Health and Disease". In Astrid Sigel, Helmut Sigel and Roland K. O. Sigel. Interrelations between Essential Metal Ions and Human Diseases. Metal Ions in Life Sciences 13. Springer. pp. 295–320

As a tree bears fruit from radiant solar power it sweetens to a nutritious level that is its highest level. Within your body a sweetness from the minerals of the fruit combine with solar power to sweeten in a fermentation of life and energy to produce energy that heals and is the power of natural healing.

This protein is important and it takes enzyme action with bacteria and a non-nucleus archaeon that use sunlight to energize and this is a natural stimulation not an inhibiting blockage of nature as artificial sweeteners do in energy drinks. These drinks of pseudo energy drinks use high concentration of fructose to excite nervous reaction that causes brain activity as cocaine.

The body is a highly complex chemical electrical system that science has just begun to understand mainly through the discovery of endocrines secretions to replicate for natural pain relievers based in opioids. Valium is the serotonin receptors that the body uses to reward for a good meal. So eat nutritious and you will give energy and bliss.

It seems so simplistic and makes perfect sense that what people have been saying that our body and mind is well served by nature. We feel this because inside we know it is the truth.

Energy speaks to us and that is what we need. Energy is within and without us and the uninhibited flow of this is what nutrition does the best and with it your health will flourish. When you see a tree and the fruit it bears and understand that your body is the same energy cycle of solar power and sugar producing from consumption for energy to burst with color then you begin to understand the connection we have to nature.

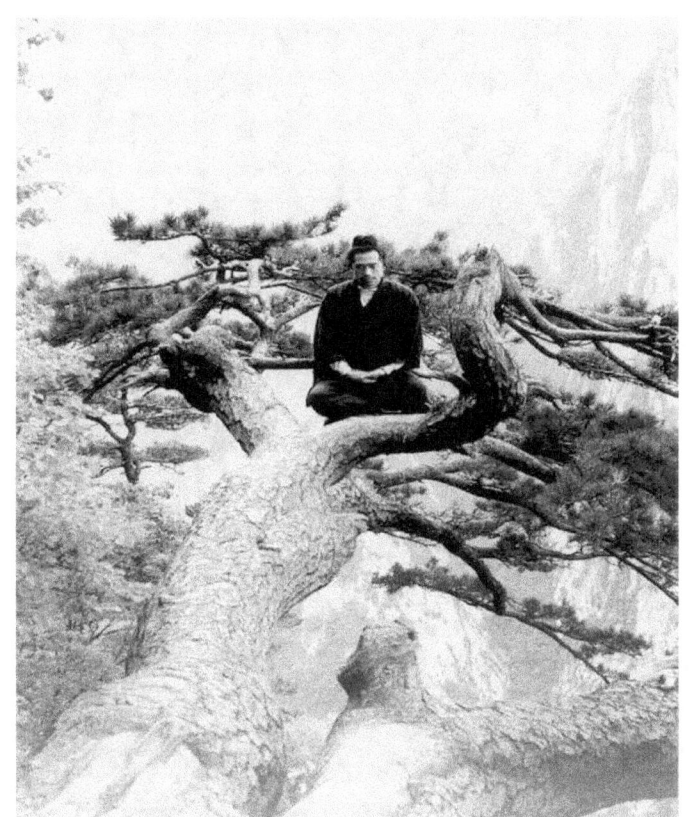

www.ingramcontent.com/pod-product-compliance
Lightning Source LLC
Chambersburg PA
CBHW081220280526
45787CB00006B/2464